About

William H. Lee, cist, nutritional researcher, master herbalist and the nutritional columnist for *American Druggist* magazine. He is the author of a number of books in the health field, including *Raw Fruit and Vegetable Juices and Drinks* and most recently, with Lynn Lee, *Herbal Love Potions.*

Lynn Lee, CN is a certified nutritionist, herbalist, and William Lee's wife and partner.

Keats Titles of Related Interest

Herbal Love Potions
William H. Lee, R.Ph., D.Sc. and
Lynn Lee, CN

The Herb Tea Book
Dorothy Hall

Creating Your Herbal Profile
Dorothy Hall

Guide to Medicinal Plants
Paul Schauenberg and Ferdinand Paris

The Bach Flower Remedies
Edward Bach, M.D. and F. J. Wheeler, M.D.

Handbook of the Bach Flower Remedies
Dr. Phillip M. Chancellor

Growing Herbs as Aromatics
Roy Genders

Daniel Mowrey Herbal Titles
Next Generation Herbal Medicine
Scientific Validation of Herbal Medicine
Proven Herbal Blends

The Book of
Practical
Aromatherapy

Including Theory and Recipes
for Everyday Use

William H. Lee, D.Sc., R.Ph.
and
Lynn Lee, CN

Authors of *Herbal Love Potions*

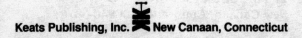

Keats Publishing, Inc. ✦ **New Canaan, Connecticut**

The Book of Practical Aromatherapy is not intended as medical advice. Its intent is solely informational and educational. Please consult a health professional should the need for one be indicated.

THE BOOK OF PRACTICAL AROMATHERAPY

Copyright © 1992 by William H. Lee and Lynn Lee

Library of Congress Cataloging-in-Publication Data

Lee, William H.
   The book of practical aromatherapy : including theory and recipes for everyday use / William H. Lee and Lynn Lee.
     p.   cm.
   Includes bibliographical references.
   ISBN 0-87983-539-7 : $4.95
   1. Aromatherapy.   I. Lee, Lynn, C.N. II. Title.
RM666.A68L44 1992
615'.321—dc20   91-34890
                                 CIP

Printed in the United States of America

Published by Keats Publishing, Inc.
27 Pine Street (Box 876)
New Canaan, Connecticut 06840-0876

Contents

Preface

Although you do not know it, you have practiced aromatherapy many times in your life:

- When you sucked on a throat or cough lozenge that contained menthol and the soothing vapors helped you feel better and opened your nasal passages.
- When your mother applied Vicks Vaporub to your chest.
- When you put perfume behind your ears and on your pulse spots to attract that certain guy.
- When you smell apple pie and you remember the way your grandmother looked when she took a hot pie from the oven.

All of the above are part of aromatherapy but there's so much more.

There's an entire discipline based on the essential oils found in the plant kingdom and the way they affect your sense of smell and touch, and even the way you think and feel.

The essential oils—sometimes called volatile oils or plant essences—can be inhaled, massaged into the skin, placed in bathwater, or even taken internally. They are healing and antiseptic and can help allay anxiety, relieve depression and contribute to a romantic evening.

This book is an introduction to the art and science of plant essences. Your world will never be the same again.

Chapter One

~~~~~~~~~~~~~~~~~~~~~~~~~~~

The Ancient Art of Aromatherapy

The Origins of Aromatherapy

Herbology, the parent form of aromatherapy, probably began when the first primitive cave-mom ate the first primitive dandelion and found that it helped to relieve her primitive PMS by ridding her body of excess fluid. That would be about 50,000 years ago.

Aromatherapy is only about 5,000 years old.

There are records in the Bible of the use of plants and their oils to treat various illnesses and volumes of information in Egyptian papyrus. In fact, the Egyptians were the first to perfect the art.

Although embalming is a dying art (no pun intended) and many of the secrets have been lost, a lot of the other formulas for health and beauty have been investigated and brought up to date. In this book you will find and be able to make some of these formulas for yourself. They have as much practical use today as they did for ancient households.

The actual study of aromatherapy probably really began when man learned to use fire. By trial and error throwing aromatic branches on the fire he began to note that certain burning branches made him feel good, others made food taste better, and still others killed the ever-present fleas. As he experimented further he discovered smoke that make him feel invigorated and smoke that made him sleepy. Of course, this had to be a gift of the gods, and soon burning aromatic wood became a ceremony.

As time passed man found that oil could be pressed from plants. The oil was pleasant when rubbed into the skin and hair but it had a drawback . . . it turned rancid and smelled bad. Then some extra-bright person discovered that a combination of oil and aromatic wood felt good and smelled nice for a much longer time and a perfume unguent was born.

However, it was not until the Egyptians put their inventive minds to work that the first real era of aromatherapy began. While the Chinese were perfecting acupuncture, the Egyptians were perfecting the art of using essential oils. The papyri records document their use in medicine, cosmetics and massage. The Ebers papyrus, dating from the 18th Dynasty, lists myrrh as an anti-inflammatory agent. It still is listed in modern texts on pharmacognosy for the same purpose. Although we rarely see a prescription for it today because doctors are not taught about it, here is the prescription for a cosmetic face pack from that papyrus:

Facial 〰〰〰〰〰〰〰〰

incense (frankincense)
myrrh
fresh oil
cypress berries

Crush the berries and mix together with the other ingredients. Stir into fresh milk and apply to the face for six days.

The priests had the aromatherapy concession and made the most of it as the first aromatics were used in the temples as offerings. Then, as shipments of various oils began to arrive from other countries, public display of ceremonies began. At the base of the Sphinx at Giza there is a tablet made of granite showing King Thutmose (1425-1408 B.C.) offering incense and libations of oil to a god with the body of a lion.

As more and more aromatics poured into Egypt, the excess products spread to the physician and to the cosmetician with a considerable increase in wealth to those who became versed in their use.

During the 1,500 years following the 18th Dynasty the Egyptians perfected their knowledge of the medicinal properties of aromatics, of perfumery, and of the making of scented unguents. There was not a clear distinction between medicines and perfumes and one item often served both purposes. The aromatics used included myrhh, frankincense, cedarwood, origanum, bitter almond, spikenard, henna, juniper, coriander, calamus and many other plants. Fumigation had its start in the ancient city of Tel-el-Amarna, where they set fire to stacks of aromatic plants in public squares to purify the air.

A mixture of 16 ingredients called *kuphi* was used as a perfume, an antiseptic and an anti-inflammatory when taken internally. This preparation was adopted later on by the Greeks and Romans as one of their most potent medicines. Plutarch said its use lulled one to sleep and allayed anxieties.

(Sounds like something we could use in today's stressful world.)

The Babylonians also used aromatics. A clay tablet from Babylon dated about 1800 B.C. is an order for oil of cedar, myrrh and cypress. This suggests that the trade in oils began at least 4,000 years ago.

The Jewish peoples began their exodus from Egypt around 1240 B.C. and their journey to the Promised Land took 40 years. Shortly after they started, Moses was given a number of commandments by the Lord, including how to make a holy oil and a holy incense. The holy oil was used to consecrate Aaron and his sons conferring on them perpetual priesthood from generation to generation. The formula consisted of what was called stacte, onycha, galbanum and frankincense. However, in this case *perfume* is meant in its original sense from the Latin *per* (through) and *fumum* (smoke), that is to say incense.

The Greeks learned about aromatics from the Egyptians. Herodotus and Democritus visited Egypt in the 4th century B.C. during the period that the Egyptians became masters of the art of floral extraction and brought much of the knowledge and techniques back with them. The Greeks ascribed a divine origin to all aromatic plants and attributed the invention of perfume to the gods.

The recipes for a number of medicinal perfumes are inscribed on marble tablets both in the temples of Aesculapius, a Greek god of healing, and the temples of Aphrodite.

The Romans were even more lavish in their use of perfume than the Greeks. They used three types of perfume: solid perfumed ointments, scented oils and powdered perfumes. These were used to scent their hair, their bodies, their clothes, their beds and even their flags.

When Rome fell, surviving Romans took refuge in Constantinople, taking their knowledge of perfumery with them. Their knowledge blended with the Byzantine expertise and trade in aromatic spices became an important factor in the known world.

It was not until the late part of the 10th century that distillation extraction was discovered (or rediscovered—no one can say for sure) by an Arabian physician known as Avicenna. It was this process that enabled perfumers to obtain pure essences. Avicenna chose the rose to experiment with and the results were so gratifying that rose water perfume soon was manufactured in quantity and the new process was applied to other plants and flowers.

The distilled products caught on in Europe and as the crusaders brought back samples, Europeans began their own perfumeries. By the end of the 12th century there was a thriving perfume business.

A number of English manuscripts from the 14th and 15th centuries contain references to herbal oils and how to make them.

Distillation and infusion were explained in detail.

In 1660 the herbalist and astrologer Nicholas Culpeper published a book especially for women detailing remedies for problems that plagued them then . . . and now.

To Make The Breasts Decrease Or Grow Less ~~~~~~~~~~

The juice of hemlock mixt with camphor and layd on makes them less; also white frankincense with navel-wort and sharp vinegar hinders their growth.

To Make Hair Grow Again ~~~

Take oyl of juniper, oyl of nuts, each one ounce, white honey, juice of dock, each half an ounce, smallage seeds, asarabacca powdered, each two ounces, incorporate them and anoint the place.

By 1900 essential oils were being used copiously by physicians. It was the golden age of herbs, but it was not to last. Louis Pasteur had found the means to vanquish bacteria and science rushed to the new medicine, relegating herbs to the back shelf and to the few who still believed.

So aromatherapy languished in obscurity until there was an accident. Freud says there is no such thing as an accident but here's what happened:

In the early 1900s, René-Maurice Gattefossé, a French chemist, was conducting experiments on the cosmetic use of essential oils. There was a small explosion in the lab and one of his hands was badly burned. In extreme pain, he plunged his hand into a bowl of what he thought was water.

Almost instantly the pain was relieved and the hand healed at an astonishing rate of speed, leaving no scar.

What he thought was water was essence of lavender, the distilled essential oil of the lavender flower.

And so began the rebirth of essential oils as medicines as well as perfumes. Gattefossé published his first book, *Aromathérapie*, in 1928 and is credited with coining the word aromatherapy. In spite of interest in this "new" medicine, the times were not fertile and the second World War buried his research.

All was not lost, however, just forgotten.

Then Jean Valnet, a French medical doctor who had always been interested in using herbs therapeutically, no doubt inspired by Gattefossé's research, began to use essential oils in his practice. He soon realized that he had a therapy with enormous potential.

In 1964 he published *The Practice of Aromatherapy* and it is almost entirely due to his work that aromatherapy is now being recognized as a therapy in its own right.

Although other countries have produced some notable researchers, for example, Drs. Gatti and Cajola of Italy, it remained for the French to bring aromatherapy to the United States. We are indebted to people like Marcel F. Lavabre who brought his knowledge of aromatherapy to the U.S. and is promulgating the use of natural essences.

Dr. Kurt Schnaubelt of the Pacific Institute of Aromatherapy in San Rafael, California is a scientist who is very familiar with the effects of plant substances on the human body. He notes that at least 40 percent of the drugs sold in his native Germany come from plant material or are composed completely of plant material, unlike the U.S., where synthetic drugs have taken over the pharmaceutical industry.

"Although it wasn't called aromatherapy back then, that's exactly what we were doing. It's important that people realize there is much more to this field than New Age jargon, 'feel good' experiences and talk of vibrations," Dr. Schnaubelt adds.

In his years of work in chemistry and as a doctor of natural sciences, he's gathered extensive documentation into the healing powers of plants from a variety of sources, including medical journals and the fields of ethnobotany, popular science and plant pharmacognosy, which he now passes on to naturopaths, homeopaths and other medical practitioners through the Pacific Institute's courses and other services.

Schnaubelt is also a staunch advocate of regulation in this burgeoning industry in the U.S., warning practitioners and consumers alike of misleading labels, product claims and questionable safety practices in his column in Common Scents, the quarterly journal of the American Aromatherapy Association.

Besides the beneficial physical and psychological effects of aromatherapy, he believes that "taking more responsibility for our own health" is "one of the most positive and fascinating aspects of aromatherapy."

Can aromatherapy help you? You won't know until you try it.

Chapter Two

~~~~~~~~~~~~~~~~~~~~~~~~~~~~~~~~

How to Use Aromatherapy to Enhance Your Life and Health

What are Essential Oils?

Essential oils aren't oily. They won't leave a grease spot on paper or cloth. They can't be used for cooking.

Essential oils are present in nature. They are the hormones of the plant. They attract insects so they can carry on sexual reproduction. They create shields against predators. They make the fragrance that attracts the bee and the sweetness that lures the hummingbird.

Does that sound like peanut oil or olive oil?

Essential oils are the heart and pulse of the plant and are present in very small amounts, sometimes as little as .01 percent. It is the plant's life force that is tapped in aromatherpay and each oil has its own unique effect upon the body and/or the mind.

We made the comparison between the essential oil and hormones because the hormones we produce in our bodies (and without which we couldn't live), are present in minute amounts also. All of the hormones coursing through us at one time would fill only a thimble. Similarly, it would take at least 10 large buckets of orange blossoms to extract a mere thimbleful of the essential oil called neroli. And, just as our glands produce various hormones which affect our bodily systems, so the plant hormones are capable of giving different effects when used correctly.

Essential oils contain a number of complex biochemicals including vitamins, antibiotics in a natural state and antiseptics. Because oils from different plants have different virtues, it's wise to learn a bit about them before you use them.

Is It Called Aromatherapy Because It Only Works Through the Nose?

The practice of using essential oils is called aromatherapy because it is the essential oil which is responsible for the fragrance in the plant kingdom. But essential oils are also used in inhalations, massage, and even internally to obtain the healing and beautifying effects.

Of course, the sense of smell plays a very important role in this artful science because the area of the brain that responds to odors is very close to the most primitive part of our brain, the part that goes furthest back to our past. This is called the limbic brain or reptile brain and it controls the way we act and react sexually and aggressively, and it influences hunger and thirst. In a way the olfactory nerve goes directly from the nose to deep in the brain, almost a direct entrance to our emotions, and once an "odor memory" is in place it's almost impossible to get rid of.

For example, say your mother wore a certain scent when she held you in her arms as a tiny babe. You will forever associate that scent with warmth, love, and protection.

Similarly, if you felt that way about your dad in your childish illusion and he wore a scented after-shave, the man in your adult life may have won your favor simply by using the same scent!

The sense of smell is a powerful tool. Imagine if there was something wrong with your sense of smell. Don't laugh, it can have disastrous results.

When the olfactory nerve is stimulated, the signals it conveys affect the digestive system, the sexual system, and the behavioral system.

We are all familiar with the operation of the nose when confronted with a strange odor. After a while it becomes "blind" to it, shuts off the external smellability so you no longer are aware that the smell is present. But the brain keeps on reacting to the odor whether you are still consciously smelling it or not. So, even when you are unaware of an odor's effect, you may still be "pushed" by its presence.

Suppose you couldn't smell anything but your brain reacted to odors anyway?

There is a condition known as *anosmia* which is the total inability to smell anything. As you can imagine, when an individual is diagnosed with this condition it is usually accompanied by severe depression.

Are there people who are more sensitive to smells than others? Sure, but they can have rewards as well as pitfalls. Consider the other extreme, the person suffering from *parosmia* or olfactory illusion. This person perceives bad odors even when they don't exist.

The sufferers from this condition relate to it in one of two ways. If they are shy and introverted they assume the bad smell originates in them. That leads to frequent baths, overuse of deodorants and perfumes and isolation.

But when a paranoid individual suffers this condition he assumes the bad smell originates with others and the smell is a warning that they are plotting against him.

The so-called Spider King, King Louis XI of France, appears to have been such a victim. He filled the prisons with people who had revealed their attempts to harm him through their evil odors. Of course they all confessed after excruciating torture so the king was proven right after all!

Our sense of smell is a leftover from our evolutionary past and is still very sensitive. It is so acute that we can detect one part of an aroma in 10,000 billion parts of air. If that something smells like a rose, we say it is a rose. This does not mean that the brain uses the same type of logic as our intellect. We are not sure exactly how our brain reacts when our intellect says it smells like a rose.

In fact, that is one reason why only natural scents are used for aromatherapy. The *nose* can be fooled by synthetic aromas but not the *brain*. In one experiment, volunteers were connected to an EEG (electroencephalogram) machine and allowed to smell synthetic rose and natural rose. They could not tell one from the other, but their brain waves showed different patterns when exposed to natural and synthetic rose.

Maybe that's why the most expensive perfumes try to use some natural substance like civet, musk, castoreum from the scent glands of animals, or at least a natural substance with elements similar to human pheromones. Sandalwood, for example, has a chemical structure similar to androsterol, a human male pheromone.

We humans secrete musky molecules. We all have been exposed to these molecules while in our mother's womb. Therefore, we may be predisposed to be attracted to these molecules after birth.

Sigmund Freud considered the repression of smell a major cause of mental illness and speculated that the nose was a sexual organ as important as the penis. Certainly, the sense of smell can make sex more exciting and even help initiate sexual contact.

Why all the emphasis on smell?

Because when you learn more about essential oils you'll learn how to influence yourself and others in the direction you wish to go.

That may be towards the bedroom.

Or towards a better mood.

Or to alleviate a hangover or jet lag.

Or to clear a stuffy office of food, chemical and tobacco odors.

All of the above can be easily accomplished through the safe and sane use of essential oils.

Okay, I'm Interested. How Do They Extract These Oils?

Before distillation there was *hand expression*.
That's squeezing!

Assuming that you are an adult—because this experiment is not to be tried by a youngster—get a candle and some fresh orange peel. Light the candle and then squeeze the peel between your fingers so the oil is released in a fine spray towards the flame.

Watch the fireworks.

The essential oil burns in the flame of the candle. You have hand expressed the volatile oil found in the peel of an orange.

This technique is confined to the citrus family. Originally the peels were squeezed by hand until the oil glands burst. The oil was collected in a sponge which was squeezed into a container when saturated.

(This was some job back in the early days before machines were invented to do the squeezing.)

Lemon, lime, mandarin orange and bergamot are obtained in this manner.

Enfleurage was the method used for extracting essential oil from flowers and is started by picking flower heads and placing them on a glass bed. The heads are then covered with purified fat.

The essential oils were absorbed by the fat. Then more flowers were laid on the glass bed and the same fat was spread on them. This went on and on until the fat was saturated with the essential oil. The result was called a pomade and and was often used in that state as an ointment or a perfume. Enfleurage is still used in India today to make solid perfume but usually the process is carried further. The pomade is dissolved in alcohol. The fat is insoluble in the alcohol but the essential oil is not. The resultant liquid is then carefully heated and the alcohol is driven off, leaving the oil behind.

Maceration. This method is similar to enfleurage and can still be used to prepare essential oils at home. The flowers or leaves are crushed to rupture the oil glands, then put into warm vegetable oil and placed in a warm place. The vegetable oil absorbs the essential oil and the flowers are strained off. A fresh lot of flowers or leaves are put into the same oil and the process is repeated until the oil is saturated with the fragrance.

The resultant liquid can be used for massage treatments or in making herbal creams.

Solvent Extraction. In simple terms, the flowers are covered with a solvent such as ether which extracts the essential oil. The ether, or whatever solvent is being used, is driven off leaving the oil behind in the container. It is a little more complicated than that, but basically that's how it's done.

Steam Distillation. The most modern method and the method most in use today is the method discovered by Avicenna. It makes use of the high volatility rate of essential oils plus the fact that they are mainly insoluble in water. The flowers or plant parts are placed in a container with water and the water is heated to steam. The steam carries off the essential oil into another container where the mixture is cooled. It is then easy to separate the oil from the water to obtain the purest essential oil.

The plant parts which can be used to supply essential oil can be the flower, peel, seed, root, leaf or any part of the bark. Even grass gives off essential oil.

I Understand How Fragrant Odors Have an Effect on People, and Getting a Massage Can Be Fun, But What Does the Oil Do?

The skin is the largest organ in the body. It covers and protects the body. It's waterproof, germproof unless broken, keeps the heat in and the cold out, gets rid of waste material and is attractive—most of the time—to the opposite sex.

A healthy skin reflects a healthy body and a flaky, blemished, irritable skin reflects something out of order. It could be diet, heredity, stress, too much sun or not enough. Diet correction, supplements, relieving the stressful situation, *and* aromatherapy can be of help in most situations.

The skin is waterproof, as said before, but essential oils can penetrate the skin and reach the small blood vessels called capillaries that are in the dermis, the layer under the epidermis which is the outer layer of the skin.

Once the oil has reached the capillaries it can be carried by the blood to actually do something useful beyond the pleasure of the massage. At the same time, if the right oils are used, the skin can be rejuvenated.

Sweat glands and oil glands in the skin work together to keep the surface of the skin supple and balanced. Excess sweat can dry the skin while excess oil can leave it greasy. If one type of gland is overactive or the other underactive, the result is either dry or oily skin.

Carrier Oils

Because essential oils are so concentrated, they must always be mixed into a carrier oil for use in a massage. The carrier or base oil may be any natural vegetable oil. One carrier oil that is very popular is grapeseed oil. It is very light, odorless and easily absorbed into the skin. Almond and sunflower oils are popular too. For very dry skin, or for some facial massages, wheat germ oil, avocado oil, jojoba and apricot kernel oil are often used in small quantites.

Take care if you're trying to blend your own oils, since they interact with each other in many different ways. Some essential and carrier oils can be marvelous helpers individually, but smell unpleasant in combination, and no one would want to use an oil with a scent they find offensive. The key is finding one you like, that affects you the way you want it, whether you're seeking the stimulation of an energizing oil or the tranquility of a soothing, more sedative-type mixture.

Here are some specifics on some of the best carrier oils and their characteristics:

Avocado Oil. This is a thick, heavy oil which helps preserve the blend due to its high vitamin E content. It also contains a large amount of vitamin A which makes it useful for people with skin problems. It is safe for individuals with allergies, particularly wheat allergies. Because it is so thick, it should only be about five percent of the mix.

Evening Primrose Oil. This oil is expressed from the seeds of *Oenothera biennis*, a tall plant with pretty yellow flowers. The oil is usually available in health food stores in capsule form and is used to support the body's efforts to heal skin conditions and other discomforts.

It is a useful addition to treatment oils for eczema and other dry skin conditions, and is soothing and healing in inflammatory allergic conditions.

Jojoba Oil. This is taken from a desert plant, *Simmondsia chinensis*. It is a waxy oil which, when diluted, gives the skin a silky feel and adds extra fluidity to a massage blend. Use about 10 percent of this oil in your mix. This oil is particularly useful for dry eczema. Jojoba is the plant equivalent to sperm oil taken from sperm whales, so its use helps save the lives of these wonderful creatures.

Peach or Apricot Kernel Oil. These are squeezed from the kernels of the *Prunus persica*, peach (therefore sometimes called persic oil), and *Prunus armenica*, the apricot. They are not particularly fragrant but are emollient and nutritive to the skin.

Soya Oil. Dry skin responds well to this oil, specifically if the person is allergic to wheat and/or dairy products.

Sweet Almond oil. This oil is squeezed from the seeds of the sweet almond. It has the characteristic smell of almonds, is pale yellow in color and has emollient, nutrient and softening qualities.

Wheat Germ Oil. A rich, nourishing oil which adds a deep orange color to the mix. It has a high vitamin E content and is very good for dry, cracked or mature skin. It helps prevent stretch marks and is soothing and healing in general. Use it up to 10 percent of your mix. This oil should not be used for anyone with a wheat allergy.

Grapeseed oil, sesame oil and sunflower seed oil are also used to make massage oils.

How to Make a Massage Oil

There are a number of useful formulas throughout this book, but here is a general guide to mixing any massage oil.

In general, a 2½ percent concentration is used.

This means that in each 100 cubic centimeters of liquid there will be 2.5 cc of essential oil.

Sounds like you have to learn math to make a massage oil. No way!

In pharmacy, we use a drop-to-cc ratio to work out prescriptions, so here's a shortcut to figure out the proportions.

If you wish to make two ounces of massage oil, figure 50 cc total volume. One drop is about 5 percent of a cc, so for 2½ percent, it's one drop per two cc. Therefore 25 drops of the essential oil in two ounces of carrier oil will equal 2.5 percent.

If you're making only one ounce of massage oil or 30 cc, take 15 drops of essential oil, and you'll have the correct dilution.

You can use one essential oil or more than one.

You can use one carrier oil or more than one.

This is your science and you are the scientist. The formulas given have been tested but you may decide to use more or less of the essential oil or the carrier oil depending on your own wishes.

Kids' Stuff

If you are making a massage oil for a child, the recommended dilution is 1¼ percent.

This amount is easily arrived at by cutting the adult dose in half. In other words, for a child's massage oil which will amount to one ounce (30 cc) you would use half of the adult amount of 15 drops, or 7½ drops to one ounce of carrier oil.

Simple, isn't it?

Everyday Aromatherapies

For Hair Care and Scalp Problems. Dandruff, dry hair, greasy hair, even when the kids bring home head lice—these conditions respond well to specific blends of essential oils such as thyme, sage and lavender, diluted as suggested, in carrier oil. Plus, they are completely natural remedies. This means that those people who react badly to chemical means are often able to use natural scents to solve their difficulties.

As a bonus . . . these treatments smell good!

Facial Creams, Lotions, Toners. In general, essential oils possess a number of therapeutic qualities which can be of extreme value.

Lavender, neroli, and patchouli, among others, have the ability to naturally stimulate skin growth and appear to have a rejuvenating effect on the skin.

Many of the essential oils are antiseptic and fight infectious germs. Other oils have an astringent cleansing effect and can be included in your formula if needed.

Sensitive skin responds well to rose and neroli which are anti-inflammatory while sandalwood and cypress help treat broken veins.

The carrier oils avocado and wheat germ, with their high vitamin content, make useful additions to help mature, cracked or dry skin.

Skin tone improves with better circulation and toxins are eliminated more easily when essential oils and massage are part of your daily life.

Inhalations, Mouthwash, Gargles. These are money-savers and better than commercial preparations because you know exactly what goes into them.

For respiratory problems and general infections, inhalations are a way of introducing the essential oil into the bloodstream. They can then stimulate the body's own defensive action to help destroy invading bacteria. The steam heat combined with oils such as eucalyptus acts on the area of infection, fighting viruses and fungi in the nose and respiratory system.

Gargles of recommended essential oils can be used to fight infections and mouthwash made with essential oils can help treat mouth ulcers, oral thrush and infected gums. To strengthen gums in particular, try fennel, lemon or sage.

Aromatic Baths. These are treats as well as treatments. They can be stimulating and refreshing in the morning or relaxing and soothing for the evening. With the right blend of essential oils such as basil or rose, they can be regenerating and sexually stimulating.

Sitz Baths. These can be useful for genitourinary infections or problems in the anal area when a recommended essential oil such as cypress is used.

Specific Treatment Formulas. For special problems such as shingles, essences can be amazingly versatile. See chapter three for specifics.

Beat the Work-Day Blues.

Waking up in the morning is one thing, wanting to get up and go to work is another.

Many of us find it difficult to start our engines in the morning. Many rely on a couple of cigarettes and four cups of coffee to get them out of the house. Not a healthy way to start the day—or live your life.

If you're that kind of person, go to the health food store today and buy tiny bottles of peppermint oil, juniper oil and rosemary oil.

Tomorrow morning you can do the following:

Jump-Starter 〰〰〰〰〰
Fill the tub halfway with warm water. Add:
5 drops rosemary oil
5 drops juniper oil
2 drops peppermint oil

Swish the water around to disperse the essences and get in and lie down. Relax for 10 minutes. Then get out, dry yourself off, eat a hearty breakfast and feel the difference you can make in your life.

After-shave lotion. Cologne. Body odor. Hair spray. Cigarette smoke. Egg salad sandwiches. Photocopy machines. The windows don't open and you face the prospect of eight hours in this stinking, stagnant, headache-making, torture chamber of a working environment.

Don't throw a chair through the nearest window and don't quit your job . . . you need the money. Use your newfound knowledge of aromatherapy to create an odor-free zone around your work area.

Keep a bottle of lemon oil, bergamot or rosewood essence in your desk drawer. When things get bad, select one of your secret weapons. Put one drop of the essential oil on each of four tissues and place one tissue at each corner of your desk.

Ah! The air will freshen in a jiffy within this fragile fortress and the antiseptic power of the essence will also help protect you from any stray bacteria floating in the air in search of a target.

Then there are times you're sitting at your desk or behind the counter wishing you were any place else but work. Nothing is cheery. You're down in the dumps and it's beginning to affect your work and your relationships with the other people around you.

What are your options? Quit? You can't. You have people depending on your salary.

Open that desk drawer and reach for the little bottle of clary sage and gently sniff at the open lip. Just a little sniff—all you want to do is get past your "down" feeling so you can finish the day. If you inhale too deeply, too often, you might get a bit high and ignore your work all together.

Just when you're looking forward to the end of the day, the boss calls you in to take his place at a meeting with a prospective account. It can mean a bonus but your mind has already begun its countdown to 5:00 p.m. You're not exactly sparkling and enthusiastic.

But you have no choice, so it's into the aromatherapy drawer. This time, go for the bottle of basil essence. Put a drop on a tissue. A sniff or two will refresh you enough for the boss to think you have a spare dynamo. It's better than three cups of black coffee—and a lot easier on your nerves and your health.

Let's make the situation even worse. The boss calls you in as in the above scenario and the new client turns out to be an ex-boyfriend you dumped in an unpleasant manner. Now it's nervous stomach time as well.

How can you cope with this stomach-churning situation?

Geranium oil can soothe a troubled tummy and give you a mental lift at the same time. You can put two drops on a bit of brown sugar and swallow the mixture. Or mix the essential oil drops with a bit of honey and water and sip.

Unless you're very unusual, there are times you get home with aching feet, so achy you wish they belonged to someone else. You don't have time to lie down or even put them up on a hassock because your date will arrive within the hour, or maybe you're due at the PTA meeting.

Feet Fixer ～～～～～～～

Aromatherapy to the rescue! All you need is a basin half-filled with warm water to which you add:

5 drops juniper
2 drops rosemary
3 drops lavender

Put the basin under the table and while you're doing something to your face to get ready, slip those aching feet into the tepid water and let the mixture roll over and between your toes.

In 10 minutes you'll feel like your feet have slept all night. Massage them gently for a minute, towel dry and you're ready for a night on the town.

For High Anxiety. I hate flying . . . at least in a plane. But if you have to, you can make yourself more comfortable during the flight and afterward. First, I'll assume you've been to your health food store and have purchased an assortment of dropper bottles containing the most popular essential oils. This is your first-aid kit.

Before you go to the airport, sip a cup or two of chamomile tea. (This will make you sleepy enough to doze during the flight.)

Then scent some tissues with two drops of bergamot, one drop of nerol and one drop of chamomile essence. Put the tissues in a sealable plastic bag, the kind that zips tightly.

Before take-off and in-flight just open the bag and sniff the soothing, sleep-inducing aromas. They'll get you to your destination with a minimum of tension and anxiety.

Dispel Jet Lag. *"But I Have an Appointment When I Get to the Hotel!"*

Bath Booster

If you have a few minutes to run some warm water in a tub, add 2 drops of rosemary and 3 drops of lemongrass. This will help you overcome jet lag and give you a quick lift.

If you have only a few minutes to yourself, run some warm water in the basin and put the same oils in the water. Swish the water and inhale the aroma that rises.

If your appointment is the next day, here's a good trick to overcome jet lag and make you brilliant again:

Take a hot bath with 2 drops of lavender and 3 drops of ylang-ylang. The delightful scent and relaxing warmth leads to wonderful, dreamless sleep—and a bright-eyed, bushy-tailed morning.

(If you prepare your aromatherapy kit before you leave, you'll find it takes only a few minutes to refresh yourself for immediate action or prepare yourself for rest. The essences are much better than sleeping pills and you won't have any side effects in the morning.)

Travel Sickness. Travel sickness is the bane of civilization that has to drive, fly or float to get from here to there. Although it begins with the inner ear, it can be handled through the nose.

Once again we resort to tissues and a zip-tight plastic bag, but for this problem we use two drops each of lavender essence and peppermint essence. If the "queasies" start to attack, sniff gently.

You can get additional help by taking a capsule or two of powdered ginger half an hour before your flight or trip. It works better than given for motion sickness.

Smelly Feet. *"My Son Wears Sneakers Most of the Time and There Are Times We Wish He Would Run Away from Home."*

Smelly feet can destroy a household. Excessive sweating in sneakers will defeat most ordinary deodorizing methods but not aromatherapy!

Get a basin he can call his own.

Funky Feet Fixer 〰〰〰

Put some tepid water in a basin big enough for both feet, plus:

3 drops clary sage
3 drops lavender
4 drops cypress

Soak those offensive weapons for 15
minutes, then pat dry and use white, cotton socks.

Repeat daily or every other day until
the condition is completely under control.

"I Work So Hard During the Week That I
Have No Energy on the Weekends."

Unless you're in such an exhausted state
that you have to call your doctor, do I have
a remedy for you!

The Energizer ~~~~~~~~~~

Fill the bathtub halfway with warm water.
Add the following:

2 drops basil
4 drops geranium
2 drops hyssop

Get in and soak for 20 minutes. Soak a
washcloth in the scented water and roll
it up and tuck it behind your neck. Let
your tank fill up with energy. Then get
out and towel dry. Have a protein meal
and you'll find you can dance the night
away.

"My Husband's Get Up and Go Got Up
and Went."

Nutrition is important and so are supplements.

This sitz bath can also do the trick.

Sizzling Sitz Bath 〰〰〰〰

Get a basin big enough to be able to sit in and put in:

2 drops peppermint essence
5 drops clary sage
2 drops jasmine

Sit in the mixture for about 10 minutes. Use on alternate days until the situation is resolved.

"Every So Often I have to Entertain A Client and I Have a Bit Too Much Alcohol. What Do You Have for That?"

Any time a hangover makes you hate the sunlight, or any other light, or any human being for that matter, here's one solution:

Hangover Helper 〰〰〰〰

Fill the bathtub halfway with warm, not hot, water. Add:

2 drops fennel
3 drops juniper
2 drops rosemary

Lie back and soak.

Take a B-complex tablet, a vitamin C tablet and a glass of tomato juice with a splash of tabasco.

As you lie there with a moist washcloth under your neck, sipping your tomato juice, you'll slowly feel the hangover leave your body and go down the drain.

Chapter Three

Therapeutic Uses of Essential Oils

I am not anti-doctor. I am against delegating all health care to someone else if there is something I can do to alleviate the problem. If aromatherapy doesn't work, then it's time to investigate other means.

Unless the situation is serious or life-threatening, give nature a chance first.

Basic Formulations

Note: *The following formulas are for adults.*

In general, these are the different methods of using essential oils. When a specific formula is given it may or may not conform to the general percentages shown.

Massage Oil

$2\frac{1}{2}$% dilution. 15 drops of essence to 1 ounce of carrier oil

Inhalation

5 to 10 drops of essence to a bowl of very hot water. Cover head and bowl with a towel and inhale the vapors.

Compress

1 to 2 drops of essence to a bowl of cold, tepid or hot water according to directions. Dip a cloth just to the surface of the water so it picks up the film of floating oil. Gently apply the compress.

Facial Preparations

1% dilution (5 drops of essence to $\frac{1}{2}$ ounce of carrier.

Room Refresher ~~~~~

Spray 2½% dilution (25 drops of essence to two ounces of water)

Antiseptic fumigation ~~~~~

5% dilution (50 drops of essence to 2 ounces of water) at regular intervals. Spray the sickroom to reduce the chance of spreading the disease and to help the patient breathe better.

Aromatic Baths ~~~~~

5 to 10 drops of the essence to a tub of water. May be diluted with 1 to 2 teaspoons of carrier oil or milk.

Sitz Baths ~~~~~

5 drops of essence to 3 pints of water. May dilute oil with 1 teaspoon of carrier oil.

Aromatherapy treatment lends itself for use along with other, more orthodox or acceptable treatment. If you are being treated by a medical doctor, it's a good idea to let him or her know what you are doing so, if the improvement warrants it, medication can be lowered or stopped altogether.

Arthritis. This condition can be helped by using essences in the bath, on compresses, or with massage, or by using combinations of all three. The essences or essential oils most valuable in treating arthritis include: rosemary, coriander, lemon, juniper, cypress, eucalyptus, yarrow, chamomile, clary sage, marjoram and lavender.

For a young client in her late twenties with arthritis, massage therapist Karin Burling of Houston blended a shower gel of lemon, juniper, rosemary, birch and eucalyptus australiana. "She was surprised at how much it helped soothe the pain in her shoulders, even when she used it by herself at home days after the massage."

Asthma. Reduce the stress which is frequently a cause of asthma attacks and investigate any allergic triggers. The inhalation of antispasmodic essences such as lavender, marjoram, frankincense, clary sage or neroli can be helpful. In this instance, put a drop of the essence on a tissue instead of using a fumigation technique.

Try gentle massage on the back with chamomile to help ease an asthma attack. Inhaling the oil can help relieve the spasm in the bronchial tubes and the calming effect should help promote deeper breathing.

(Of course, if an inhaler has been prescribed by a medical doctor, it should not be discontinued. What can be done is a demonstration of the use of the essences in the doctor's office.)

Athlete's Foot and Ringworm. This condition can be treated with undiluted tea-tree oil, myrrh and lavender. Tea-tree oil and myrrh have antifungal action which can kill the infectious agent.

Use white cotton socks during treatment and for two weeks after it is cleared. Wash all socks in boiling water to kill the fungus.

Keep feet as dry as possible and try to walk barefoot when you are in your home.

Bronchitis. This condition can exist in an acute form as a result of bacterial infection or in a chronic state due to allergy, asthma or some other condition.

For the acute state, restrict the intake of dairy products and those containing refined carbohydrates. Do not smoke or be exposed to second hand smoke.

Inhalation 〰〰〰

Make an inhalation using:

3 drops tea-tree
1 drop eucalyptus
4 drops lemon
1 drop peppermint
1 drop sage

This can loosen mucus, act as a decongestant, expectorant and anti-viral and anti-bacterial agent. Use three times a day.

For a chronic condition, try an inhalation with a mixture of:

4 drops cedarwood
3 drops rosemary
3 drops eucalyptus

The mixture will help get rid of excess phlegm.

Bruises. An ice-cold compress should be applied at once. Lavender essence should also be applied immediately for an analgesic and anti-inflammatory action. Vitamin C and the bioflavonoids are also helpful.

Burns. Minor burns respond nicely to a few drops of lavender oil. This treatment helps prevent blistering, infection, scarring and will reduce pain.

Major burns require medical treatment immediately, if possible. If there is no way to get medical help, soak sterile gauze in lavender and apply to the area. Change the gauze every two hours and try to get medical help as soon as possible.

Cellulite. Some doctors say there is no such thing as cellulite but people with the dimpled fat deposits know it exists no matter what it is called. (Essence of rose by any other name would smell as sweetly.)

Drink eight glasses of water a day, stay away from refined sugar and refined carbohydrates, exercise vigorously and massage the thighs and hips with oils like rosemary, cypress, geranium, juniper and fennel. Also, aromatic baths with these essences can be helpful for stimulating the circulation in the area and removing trapped toxins.

Cold Sores. This mouth irritation is caused by the herpes simplex virus. Usually there is a stinging sensation just before the sore erupts. If you can catch it at the onset, you can prevent a full sore by applying lavender essence or tea rose immediately.

Cold Sore Remedy ∿∿∿∿

If a cold sore has already erupted, prepare the following mixture:

5 cc (1 teaspoonful) vodka
2 drops bergamot
2 drops eucalyptus
2 drops tea-tree

Dab the sore with the mixture alternating with dabs of undiluted lavender essence. The effect is antiseptic and healing.

Cystitis. This inflammation of the bladder is painful and can recur if life's stresses are not relieved. The condition should respond to antibacterial, anti-inflammatory oils. The sitz bath is preferable for this condition. Use tea-tree, sandalwood, bergamot, and chamomile essences in the dilution shown for sitz baths.

The same combination can be used as a hot-water compress if the pain is acute. Apply the compress to the abdomen.

In general, loose clothing rather than tight clothing is better as a preventive and during attacks. (If you've been looking for an excuse to throw away your pantyhose, here it is!) Also, cotton undergarments are better than synthetics.

Fatigue (also Chronic Fatigue Syndrome). In the main, your diet should consist of complex carbohydrates and vegetables. Avoid caffeine in any form. Swear off sugar, synthetic sweeteners, chocolate and nuts. Take a high-potency vitamin and mineral supplement three times a day. Take co-enzyme Q-10 (30 mg twice a day), fish oil capsules (2 with meals), L-carnitine (500 mg daily) and injections of vitamin B12 with your doctor's approval.

Baths with essences such as peppermint, rosemary, geranium, bergamot, clove, nutmeg and thyme can help revitalize you. (Do not use more than two drops of clove, thyme or nutmeg to half a tub of water.) Massage with peppermint, rosemary, geranium or bergamot to relieve tension.

Chronic fatigue syndrome is a real condition and should be brought to the attention of a nutritionally oriented health professional. Try the nutritional regimen and supplemental suggestions for 60 days and you should see results.

Flatulence. Gas, rumbles, windy blasts can be uncomfortable to say the least. Essential oils can help prevent gas formation as well as help expel it from the body.

When used as a massage, a clockwise rotation of oil on the abdomen will speed relief. The oils best suited for this condition include aniseed, tangerine, nutmeg, spearmint, peppermint, parsley, fennel, caraway and cinnamon.

Internally, a drop or two of peppermint

essence on a bit of brown sugar has been known to alleviate the distress.

Headaches. Taken internally, a capsule of the feverfew herb can help to relieve a migraine headache. It is available at health food stores.

A compress of lavender can be applied to the forehead or the back of the neck.

Massage a drop of lavender essence gently into the forehead. Use an inhalation of peppermint and lavender. Or try an inhalation with rosemary and eucalyptus (this combination is for sinus headaches in particular).

Lavender and neroli are excellent as a massage for tension headaches.

Chronic headaches could be the result of poor diet and a stressful life style but could also indicate a medical condition that requires attention from a health professional.

Hypertension. High blood pressure should be treated by a health professional. However, all natural means should contribute to lowering pressure to the individual's acceptable level. You should combine a recommended diet with exercise, supplements and regular massages with your choice of three of these essences: rosemary, hyssop, peppermint, frankincense and sage.

These stimulating herbs can influence circulation and, the better the circulation, the easier the blood can travel around the body thereby helping to lower the blood pressure level.

Indigestion. Herbal teas can be very helpful for this condition. Chamomile, fennel or peppermint are best.

Abdominal massage in a clockwise motion has been found to be helpful when these essences are used: lavender, rosemary, chamomile, marjoram.

The massage herbs have an antispasmodic action and will promote relaxation and proper digestion. As should be obvious by now, essences can penetrate the skin and reach the bloodstream to be circulated throughout the body. That's why a massage on the outside can help indigestion on the inside!

Insomnia. Sleeping pills prevent rapid eye movement and can give you a "blah" feeling in the morning. One of the amino acids, L-tryptophan, will help you get a restful sleep but, unless the FDA has okayed its sale by the time you are reading this, you can't buy it.

Essences are particularly effective in normalizing sleep patterns because they promote relaxation of body and mind. The oils used for this purpose are usually anti-depressive and sedative in action.

Use as a massage or an aromatic bath before bedtime. Lavender, neroli, clary sage, chamomile, sandalwood or frankincense can lull you to sleep in no time. You can even scent a tissue and place it near your pillow if you wake during the night.

Needless to say, avoid alcohol, coffee, tea, colas, hot chocolate and any other stimulant.

Mouth Ulcers. These painful intrusions can be the result of allergy, poor diet or the lack of certain nutrients such as the B complex and vitamin C.

For direct treatment, dry the area and dab with tea-tree essence on a cotton swab morning and night.

To speed healing, make a solution of 2 drops of tea-tree essence, 2 drops of myrrh essence and a teaspoon of salt to a glass of warm water as a mouthwash.

During the day, dab the area occasionally with essence of myrrh on a cotton swab. The dual attack should shorten the painful period.

Both tea-tree and myrrh are antiseptic in action and are particularly effective when the ulcer is due to an overgrowth of the yeast *Candida albicans*. Adding yogurt to the diet or capsules of *Lactobacillus acidophilus* can help prevent their recurrence.

Nausea. This condition has many causes, including motion sickeness, indigestion, overeating, sluggish digestion, emotional anxiety, tension and stress.

Mint oils help with motion sickness. The citrus oils aid digestion. Chamomile, lavender and neroli calm the nerves.

Lemon, mandarin, tangerine and orange have a cleansing aroma, which is very useful when one is in this green-faced, uncomfortable state.

Inhale the essences and sip tea made from chamomile, fennel, spearmint, or peppermint.

Edema. Water retention can be a problem for anyone who has to stand for long periods of time. Puffy and/or painful ankles can make your life miserable.

What you need are circulation-stimulating oils like rosemary and juniper, in a massage cream. Massage up the leg towards the heart to help get rid of excess fluids. Regular exercise and raising the legs above the heart can also help.

Herbs such as uva Ursi and buchu are available in health food stores and act as diuretics in a more gentle manner than those available on prescription.

Palpitations. Those annoying rapid heartbeats from stress and anxiety respond well to aromatic baths and massage to lessen stress.

Ylang-ylang in massage oil is very relaxing. Other essences which calm and soothe the spirit are chamomile, lavender, neroli and petitgrain. Any of these essential oils can be used as a massage or as a relaxing aromatic bath.

Diet control, gentle exercise and stress-relaxation training can help shield you against those unnerving irregular heartbeats.

Of course, you must check with your health practitioner to make sure there isn't an organic cause that requires either herbal medicine or prescription medicine. If so, aromatherapy makes a wonderful adjunct to other treatment.

Shingles. This is an eruption of acute, inflammatory vesicles on the trunk of the body, usually along a peripheral nerve path. They can be very painful.

Dab-On Soother

For small, painful blisters from shingles use undiluted equal parts of eucalyptus essence, tea-tree essence and bergamot. Apply with a cotton swab.

Extract

If there is a large area to be uncovered, use this:

20 drops eucalyptus
20 drops tea-tree essence
20 drops bergamot essence
2 ounces vodka

Mix together and pat on.

Soothing Soaks

To make a soothing bath, use the following in warm water:

2 drops eucalyptus
6 drops bergamot
2 drops tea-tree

This mixture also works wonderfully:

4 drops lavender
5 drops bergamot
1 drop chamomile

These treatments help to ease the pain, reduce inflammation, and exert an antiviral action. Lavender in particular is more helpful in the later stages since it is a general convalescent aid.

Shingles are not life-threatening but can be very painful for the sufferer and all of those around him or her.

Thrush. This is a fungal infection, caused by *Candida albicans*, of mouth or throat, characterized by formation of white patches and ulcers. It may also affect other areas such as the mucous membrane of the outer vagina where the itching may drive a woman into temporary insanity.

Make a douche of 2 drops of rose, 4 drops lavender and 2 drops bergamot to 2 pints of warm water, shake well, and use morning and night until the water returns clear. Then use once a week for a month, then stop.

Tea-tree (3 drops) can be applied to a tampon and used accordingly.

Aromatic baths using lavender, tea-tree and bergamot can be soothing.

Take yogurt or capsules of *Lactobacillus acidophilus* regularly to help overcome the chronic *Candida albicans* overgrowth that is the causative agent.

Toothache. Get to a dentist! But in the meantime, for the temporary relief of pain or a cavity, put some clove essence on some cotton and place it against the aching spot or cavity. Clove is a local anesthetic and antiseptic which will numb an area temporarily and cleanse the area of bacteria.

To help treat an abscess apply tea-tree

essence to the area on a regular basis until healed. You can also apply a hot compress of chamomile and lavender.

The compress will help ease the pain of an infection and help bring blood to the area. This removes some of the infected material and eases the pressure. Tea-tree has strong antiseptic properties and will kill the bacteria it comes in contact with.

However, these remedies should be considered temporary aids only and do not take the place of a visit to a good dentist.

Warts. Dip a silken thread into water at the stroke of midnight on a moonlit night and tie it tightly around the wart. Turn around three times while sprinkling salt over the left shoulder. Inside of a week your wart will be gone, according to folklore . . . unless the silk you used was polyester.

Why not try aromatherapy? Put a drop of lemon essence or tea-tree essence on the wart and cover it with a bandage. Reapply daily until the wart disappears. It can take up to a month to work its antiviral action and clear the wart completely, but it will work.

For Women Only

Menstrual Pain. It can't be "cured" in the conventional way that cure is used because it is a recurring symptom of a natural action. However, it can usually be helped in one way or another. Nutritional help includes the use of vitamin B6, calcium and other vitamins and minerals to be taken two weeks before the cycle begins.

Maggie Tisserand in *Aromatherapy For Women* states the way she handles her problems is by taking 3 drops of clary sage oil in honey water at the onset of her period when the pain is at its worst. She take one dose and that's all she needs.

If internal use of clary sage is not desired you might try making a massage oil using 15 drops of clary sage to 2 ounces of carrier oil and massaging the abdomen, inner thighs and lower back.

Amenorrhea. If a scanty flow is the cause of problems, aromatic baths and massage with chamomile, sage, clary sage, geranium, fennel and hyssop can promote a normal flow.

Dysmenorrhea. For the opposite problem, an abnormally heavy flow, massage and aromatic baths can be helpful along with diet, exercise and nutritional supplements which include iron. (The iron should preferably be in the form of ferrous gluconate which will not upset your stomach.) Cypress, rose and geranium have a normalizing effect.

Hot Flashes. Some women breeze through the menopausal period without a problem while others find themselves drenched with perspiration as they shift gears in later life.

The hot flashes, itching and perspiration respond well to aromatic baths and gentle massage with geranium and rose. Chamomile, lavender, neroli, petitgrain, jasmine, clary sage, sandalwood and ylang-ylang can also be helpful.

A good supplement program which includes a high-potency vitamin and mineral supplement (including calcium and magnesium, gamma linolenic acid, vitamin E and extra vitamin C) can help.

Is estrogen therapy indicated? Discuss this thoroughly with your health-care provider before making up your mind.

Mastitis. This condition used to be called "milk fever" and it can be very painful. You may also feel feverish. It can result from a clogged milk duct in the breast or from incomplete emptying of milk from the breast during nursing. Cleanliness is one important factor, as is expressing surplus milk if you want to avoid mastitis or relieve the condition. In the latter case, relief may be obtained by using a compress locally. Mix 1 drop geranium, 1 drop lavender and 2 drops rose in 1½ pints of cool water.

This helps to cool the hot feeling in the breast. This condition is one which requires the help of a professional. Aromatic baths with clary sage and lavender can be used in conjuction with professional treatment.

Postnatal Depression. It's real, not imagined, and probably due to changes in hormone levels after the birth.

When you can take a bath, scent it with a few drops of ylang-ylang or jasmine or clary sage and watch the way your depression departs.

Of course, any serious or ongoing depression should be discussed with your obstetrician as soon as possible.

Premenstrual Syndrome (PMS). Try GLA (gamma-linolenic acid) three times a day, two weeks before your period. Also extra calcium and vitamin B6.

Aromatic baths with lavender, neroli, geranium and rose will help to wash that extra tension away.

A relaxing massage with your favorite oil can also do wonders.

In general, up to five essences can be used in any combination. However, you may find that single essences can be more helpful to you. We are all individuals and react in our own unique ways. As a general rule, from one to three essences are most effective.

Pruritis. This word means itching.

It can pertain to the vagina or the anus and where there's an itch there's a problem that needs professional help.

Along with that, if it's the result of some external irritant like a deodorant or toilet water used on the genitals (bad idea, they should *never* be used there), discontinue at once. If it's caused by food or drink and you can isolate the item or items, discontinue them.

If the itch is caused by an infection, see

your doctor. However, if there's no discharge and the mucous membrane is dry and not red and irritated, try an aromatic bath with lavender and rose.

Leucorrhea. A light vaginal discharge is normal but prolonged, heavy discharge can be the sign of trouble.

The source could be a food allergy or *Candida* and you may need professional help. You could try using a douche of lavender, bergamot and rose to see if the condition is easily resolved. Add 2 drops rose, 4 drops lavender, 2 drops bergamot to 2 pints of warm water. Shake well before using.

The Properties and Uses of Essential Oils

Again, we are not suggesting that anyone try essential oils willy-nilly without the aid of a trained aromatherapist, and, although physicians in England, France, Germany and other parts of Europe do prescribe some carefully selected essential oils internally for patients under their care, none of these should ever be ingested without a doctor's supervision. The purpose of this list is to simply introduce you to the wide variety of potential uses of aromatic oils. It is by no means all-inclusive; it covers the ones which are most likely to be found.

Angelica Root. This essential oil acts as a carminative, cleanser, digestive and reviving stimulant; it also has antispasmodic qualities.

Use angelica root in cases of fluid or toxin build-up, to treat migraine headaches and digestive upsets, anemia, anorexia; for spasms of the digestive system, for gout and as a general aid for convalescents.

Aniseed. Acts as an antispasmodic, aphrodisiac, and carminative. (No wonder anisette is popular as an after-dinner liqueur!)

Try this for spasms of the digestive system and excess gas, sexual dysfunction and migraine. French doctors schooled in aromatherapy often recommend aniseed to nursing mothers, to help promote milk production.

Basil. Helps stimulate feelings and the psyche; acts as a tonic to treat nervous conditions; is a stomachic and intestinal antiseptic, and has antispasmodic properties. Often used as an aid during birth and nursing.

Try basil in cases of migraine, dyspepsia, pregnancy and nursing (the latter two only under a doctor's supervision, of course); infections of the intestines, nervous exhaustion and stress, and in cases of short-term memory loss.

Bay. Acts as an antiseptic, stimulant and analgesic; it stimulates the scalp and skin.

Use bay to promote hair growth, to help the respiratory system, against infectious diseases, neuralgia and muscle pain.

Benzoin Resinoid. Acts as a rejuvenating stimulant, especially on the skin, and is an expectorant. This essential oil is often used as a balancing agent and to regulate body systems, as an antiseptic and diuretic, and to encourage faster healing.

Use as an aid to promote circulation; against secretions, bronchitis, laryngitis and coughs; against urinary tract infections; and to help maintain young, taut skin, as well as heal dermatitis and skin wounds.

Bergamot. Some days we all could use a lift. Instead of reaching for a sugary treat or a hit of caffeine, try a little bergamot. It acts as an antidepressant and to lift the emotions. Bergamot is also a balancing stimulant; an antiseptic, especially in skin and body care; an antispasmodic and a digestive for those with tummy trouble.

Bergamot is useful in cases of acne, eczema, dandruff and other skin conditions; it fights intestinal infections, anxiety and helps in nervous system complaints. Doctors who practice aromatherapy call on this essential oil to treat leucorrhea and vaginal pruritis.

(Caution: Because bergamot increases photosensitivity, do not use on the skin before sunning.)

Birch. Acts as an analgesic, diuretic and cleanser.

Birch is useful in cases of arthritis and rheumatism, edema, cellulitis, water retention and obesity. It is also helpful in some kidney conditions and against cystitis.

Cajeput. The aromatic oil of this Australian native has been used medicinally for literally centuries. It acts as an antiseptic, especially for the intestines and the genitourinary system; and as an antispasmodic, analgesic and expectorant.

Use for disorders of the respiratory system such as asthma, bronchitis and tuberculosis; earaches and sinusitis; in infectious diseases; against cystitis and urinary tract infections, and to fight intestinal parasites and diarrhea.

Chamomile (Blue Chamomile). Acts as a soothing, anti-inflammatory healer for skin and body; it's also analgesic, soothing to the nerves and acts as a sedative.

Use to treat acne, dermatitis, eczema and for very sensitive or inflamed skin, as well as boils, abscess and bruising. Arthritics often find blue chamomile eases the pain of swollen and "hot" joints. It also relieves toothaches and teething pain, and is often used to treat colitis.

Chamomile (German). For general body and skin care, it acts as an anti-inflammatory, stimulates the immune system; has sedative and calming properties for nervous conditions, acts naturally to balance the psyche and cases of emotional upset; and is a digestive, stomachic and antispasmodic.

As do the other types of chamomile, German chamomile helps skin conditions such as acne, dermatitis, eczema, sensitive or inflamed skin. It is useful in cases of arthritis, joint inflammation, abscess or boils. European doctors well-versed in aromatherapy find German chamomile help colitis, headaches (including migraine), insomnia, irritability; amenorrhea, menopause and other disorders of the female reproductive system; anemia, digestive problems, liver congestion; and helps soothe anger.

Chamomile (Roman). Acts as a healing agent for body and skin care, soothes sensitive skin; and is an antispasmodic with calming and sedative effects.

This type of chamomile is used to treat boils and abscess; headaches (including migraine), irritability, insomnia; and disorders of the female reproductive system including amenorrhea, dysmenorrhea and menopausal symptoms. It is also called upon to treat anemia, toxic accumulations in the liver and spleen, and chronic anger, toothache and teething.

Because of its calming effects on the mind and emotions, some aromatherapists use Roman chamomile in diffusers while they meditate or pray, while massage therapists diffuse it in the air during massage to help reduce stress in their burned-out clients.

Cardamom. Acts as a stimulant and has some aphrodisiac properties.

The essential oil of cardamom is useful in cases of impotence, as well as diarrhea and other digestive disorders.

Carrot Seed. Acts as a cleanser and tonic for the body and skin, and has stimulating properties.

Try carrot seed for cases of dermatitis, sagging, wrinkled or sun-damaged skin; and to help eliminate excess fluid and toxins from the body. Carrot seed also gives a boost of natural energy, acts as a tonic on all the glands; and helps amenorrhea, dysmenorrhea and premenstrual syndrome.

Cedarwood. Acts as an antiseptic and fungicidal, as a general tonic and for skin and scalp care.

It is also used to treat hair loss, eczema, dandruff and greasy hair; to promote relaxation (cedarwood is sometimes used in a diffuser during yoga sessions) and alleviate stress and anxiety. This potent essential oil even fights fungal infections, cystitis and urinary infections, and ulcers.

Cinnamon Bark. Acts as a stimulant, antiseptic, antispasmodic and aphrodisiac.

Aromatherapists find it promotes good circulation through the heart and central nervous system; fights influenza, intestinal infections and other infectious diseases; helps in cases of impotence, and as an aid during childbirth; and is useful against parasitic infestations like lice and scabies.

(Caution: Don't use in a concentrated form on the skin, because it will cause irritation. Too much taken internally may cause convulsions, which is why internal use of essential oils is never recommended except under a doctor's direction.)

Citronella. Yes, this is the essential oil that candles and torches made for outdoors contain. Citronella acts as a deodorant, deodorizer and purifer; it repels insects and is antiseptic and stimulating.

Citronella was used during epidemics in years past. It also helps to promote sanitation in the bathroom and where garbage containers are housed; and it is helpful against infectious diseases and for digestive disorders.

Clary Sage. Used in many body care products, clary sage acts to regenerate skin cells and is very soothing. It also regulates scaling or flaky skin and stimulates the scalp. Medicinally clary sage is used as an antispasmodic and tonic, and is valued for its antidepressant qualities.

Try this essential oil for wrinkled and aging skin, to regulate oily or overly dry skin or hair, and to promote new hair growth. Doctors trained in aromatherapy use clary sage to treat menstrual problems such as cramps and premenstrual syndrome, amenorrhea and dysmenorrhea; it's also helpful in cases of tension, anxiety and postnatal depression.

Clove Buds. Talk about something for everyone! Clove buds act as a stimulant, antiseptic, analgesic, carminative, stomachic, aphrodisiac and sharpen the intellect.

Ever try oil of cloves on a painful tooth? That's a form of aromatherapy. Clove relieves toothache, neuralgia and muscle pain, as well as helping heal urinary infections and infectious diseases, particularly those of the respiratory system. Also useful against impotence, brain fatigue and poor memory.

Cypress. This essential oil has a number of medicinal uses, including as an overall tonic and circulatory aid, as an astringent, an antispasmodic and even as a deodorant/deodorizer.

Try a whiff of cypress to lift sagging energy and help your respiratory system. Medical practitioners use it to treat cellulitis, edema, water retention, excess perspiration of the hands and feet, and in cases of chronic or whooping cough, even asthma.

Eucalyptus. As with chamomile, there are several varieties of eucalyptus. Generally it is used medically as an antiseptic and to kill harmful bacteria, as an expectorant, and to stimulate and restore balance to body systems.

It is most often called upon to treat infectious diseases or used in a diffuser to kill germs in a sick room (in France, many hospitals use this essential oil). Some varieties are used to treat chronic sinus problems and even diabetes.

Everlasting. This essential oil is considered a wonderful asset by practitioners of aesthetic aromatherapy because of its effect on the skin and body. It has anti-inflammatory and soothing properties, as well as being an astringent and healing stimulant.

People with acne, dermatitis, inflamed or sensitive skin find everlasting helps heal all these conditions. Medical practitioners have used this aromatic oil to heal abscesses, boils and skin wounds of all kinds. It also acts beneficially on the liver and spleen.

Fennel. This essential oil is also called upon to care for the skin and body because of its cleansing and detoxifying action. It revives and stimulates the body's own healing process, acts as a carminative, antispasmodic, and digestive.

Salons use fennel to fight cellulite, fat deposits that resemble "orange-peel skin" on the thighs and derrière and plague both women and men. Because it helps eliminate excess fluids and toxins from the body, fennel is considered an aid in treating obesity and edema. It also regulates the female reproductive system, and is used to treat amenorrhea, dysmenorrhea and premenstrual syndrome.

(Caution: This essential oil is potent and, like most of the essential oils discussed in this book, should never be used on young children except under a doctor's supervision.)

Frankincense. As it was during the time of Christ, frankincense is still considered a precious substance by aromatherapists. Besides its qualities as a cooling, drying tonic and system balancer, it is antiseptic (especially for chest and lung conditions) and is an expectorant. Aromatherapists also value this essential oil for its effects on the psyche and mind. Some even consider it an aid in enhancing psychic abilities.

Frankincense is used to treat wrinkled skin, inflammation, infected wounds, asthma, lung disorders and catarrh.

Geranium. This lovely-to-look-at plant has other beneficial qualities, many of which come from its aromatic oil. The multi-faceted essential oil is often used in body and skin care because it has cell-regenerating (cytophylactic), antiseptic and astringent properties. It is also a regulator which can help diabetics and others with conditions where a system in the body is out of whack, including problems with the adrenal glands, such as occur with allergy. Geranium is also a natural insect repellant (mosquitoes in particular dislike it) and acts positively on the emotions.

Aromatherapy salons use geranium to treat clients with acne and oily skin, those with chronic or nervous skin rashes, and to revive aging skin. It is also used to fight infectious diseases, sore throats and tonsillitis, and to heal wounds, including burns. Geranium also helps the kidneys and those with kidney stones and is a diuretic. People suffering from depression or anxiety often find this essential oil helps lift their oppressive moods.

Ginger Root. This plant has an ancient history, especially in Chinese medicine and herbology. The essential oil is valued for its stimulating, antiseptic, analgesic, astringent, antispasmodic and even aphrodisiac properties. It is even reputed to help sharpen the mind and soothe the emotions.

Try a little ginger root for impotence or other sexual dysfunction, or a faulty memory. It is a digestive aid that also helps gastric spasms, excess gas and diarrhea. The essential oil also cools down fevers, nips migraines in the bud, and can help make arthritics more comfortable.

Grapefruit. Citrus fruits produce valuable essential oils and this refreshing plant is no exception. Grapefruit is both stimulating and acts to drain the body of excess secretions, including acting as a diuretic. (Perhaps this is where grapefruit first got its reputation as a dieter's best friend.)

Practitioners rely on this aromatic oil to drain and regulate the lymph system, help in digestive disorders, cellulitis, and obesity.

Jasmine. Many people find the scent of jasmine very sensual and stimulating, and one of its medicinal uses is as an aphrodisiac. It is prized in body and skin care products for its moisturizing and soothing properties, especially on dry or sensitive skin.

Jasmine also has antidepressant properties, which are often tapped in cases of chronic anxiety, postnatal depression, or times of sadness.

Juniper. Acts as a tonic and cleanser, especially in skin and body care products. Because it helps promote lymphatic drainage, juniper is helpful in cases of acne and dermatitis.

European physicians rely on its antiseptic and diuretic effects to treat some urinary infections, diabetes, rheumatism and arthritis.

Lavender. The essential oil of this plant has been used literally for centuries as an antiseptic, cytophylactic healer. But it has many other qualities as well. It is antispasmodic, acts as a gentle calmer, can help balance abnormal menstruation, and is a decongestant.

Use lavender to treat acne and oily skin, eczema, dermatitis and to soothe and help heal psoriasis. Wounds, bruises and abscesses respond well to this plant. Medical practitioners use lavender to treat asthma, bronchitis, colds, chronic sinus conditions and menstrual and menopausal disorders. It can also help migraine headaches and even insomnia.

Lavender even repels fleas and moths, which may account for its old-fashioned use as a fragrant sachet in drawers and closets.

Lemon. Acts as an astringent and refreshing tonic, a natural deodorizer and deodorant, and an antiseptic, viricidal agent and disinfectant. Lemon also helps stimulate the immune system and can perk up depressed psyches.

Use lemon to fight oily or blotchy skin, and to fight off germs and viruses.

Lemongrass. This is yet another of Nature's disinfectants, deodorants, insect repellants and deodorizers. Its astringent and tonic action helps open pores and stimulates healing. Lemongrass also acts as a digestive and stomachic.

Use to promote sanitation, fight off mosquitoes, to calm digestive system woes and prevent infections.

(Caution: Lemongrass may irritate the skin and should not be directly applied in a concentrated form.)

Lime. The oil from the peel of this tartly refreshing fruit is a natural tonic, stimulant, digestive and antispasmodic. It is also antiseptic and acts as a lymphatic system drainer.

Lime is especially useful in cases of digestive and liver problems, gall bladder symptoms, obesity and water retention. It also helps drain catarrh and eases asthma and bronchial problems, and has long been used as a general aid in convalescence because of its mildly uplifting aspects.

Marjoram. There are a number of medicinal uses for marjoram. It is an antispasmodic (calming digestive and respiratory spasms), a sedative, a vasodilator, a digestive and an analgesic.

It can be used to treat menstrual problems (including premenstrual syndrome), high blood pressure, arthritis and migraines. Nervous tension and insomnia also respond to marjoram.

Melissa. An antiseptic, stimulant and cytophylactic viricide, melissa also acts as a natural antidepressant.

Use to treat eczema, dermatitis and acne; to stimulate the metabolism, fight viruses, and ease symptoms of grief, shock and stress.

Mugwort. This essential oil sounds like something that would be featured in a witch's arsenal, and in ages past, it probably was. Besides treating toothache and the pain of teething, mugwort is often called upon to treat "'female problems" including premenstrual syndrome, and menopausal symptoms and irregularities.

Some aromatherapists believe mugwort can stimulate and help people tap into their hidden psychic powers.

Neroli. The overall effect of this fragrant essence is calming and soothing. It's used as a sedative and to ease palpitations, hysteria and anxiety.

Neroli often appears in many body and skin care formulas for its healing and calming effect on sensitive skin.

Nutmeg. In the U.S. the odor of nutmeg is most often associated with Thanksgiving and winter feasts, but did you know that it has aphrodisiac qualities as well? Nutmeg is used medicinally as an analagesic, an antiseptic, a carminative and a stimulant.

Physicians use nutmeg to treat digestive disorders and flatulence, muscle pains and neuralgia, rheumatism and nervous fatigue.

(Caution: High doses of nutmeg—even in its seemingly innocuous form as a spice for cooking—can be dangerous.)

Orange. Acts as a stimulant, especially of the lymph system, a digestive and a sedative.

Used to treat water retention, obesity, digestive symptoms and heart palpitations. Because of its sedative properties, orange is sometimes used to treat hysteria, stress and chronic insomnia.

Oregano. This is used medicinally as a stimulant, a viricide, to fight toxins, an antiseptic, antispasmodic and rubefacient. (And you thought it only made Italian food taste great!)

Helps treat the respiratory system, fights viruses, is used to treat asthma, catarrh and bronchitis, boosts circulation.

(Caution: Never use in a concentrated form directly on the skin, since it can be very irritating.)

Patchouli. Because of its popularity as a scent during the hippie era of the late sixties, I used to refer to this irreverently as "eau de rock concert." However, patchouli has many uses as a tool of medicine, especially in body and skin care. It acts as a decongestant, a fungicide, and stimulates the growth of healthy tissue.

Used to treat dermatitis, eczema, acne, chapped or wounded skin, seborrhea and impetigo—even dandruff and certain fungal conditions. It also exerts a calming effect on anxious persons.

Peppermint. Acts as an antiseptic, antispasmodic, decongestant, stomachic and digestive, an antidepressant and an analgesic. Peppermint is considered an aphrodisiac in some ancient cultures.

Useful in treating dermatitis and acne, imbalances of the metabolism, prevents the spread of infectious diseases, soothes and opens up the sinuses, eases the pain of headaches (including migraine). As a nervous system stimulant it can be used to treat vertigo and fainting spells. It also lowers fevers and helps many digestive problems including nausea and vomiting.

A whiff of peppermint will often fend off mental fatigue and give you a lift when you are working late on an important project.

Pine. It's no accident Madison Avenue jumped on the pine bandwagon for use in household cleaning products. Pine is antiseptic, especially in the urinary tract, acts as an expectorant, and is a warming tonic for the body.

Pine is used to treat colds, sore throats and other respiratory problems, genitourinary system complaints and infections, and also has a slight sedative action which makes it soothing to the nerves.

Rose. One of the most prized and costly of all the essential oils, rose is also extremely useful. Because of its ability to promote cell regeneration, it appears in many skin and body care formulas. Rose is also a natural moisturizer, regulates many body systems, is astringent and stimulating (including having some aphrodisiac properties).

Use to treat aging and wrinkled skin, sensitive and dry skin, and eczema. Also used for disorders of the reproductive system, and to give a lift during times of sadness or grief.

Rosemary. Acts as a tonic on the heart and entire cardiovascular system. It is also antiseptic, cytophylactic, antispasmodic, analgesic (especially for muscle pain) and a stimulant.

Use to treat dermatitis, acne, dry skin, eczema; also bronchitis and asthma; anemia and overall debility; arthritis and rheumatism.

Sandalwood. The aura of the East permeates this soothing essential oil, which acts as a healing moisturizer, an antiseptic and as an antidepressant.

Use sandalwood to treat and soothe troubled and chapped skin, against cystitis, to give a lift during dark and gloomy moods; and, as an aid to meditation, diffuse the essential oil in the air.

Savory. Acts medicinally as an antibiotic, antiseptic, analgesic, rubefacient and stimulating tonic.

Fights infectious disease, anemia, rheumatism and arthritis.

(Caution: Using in a concentrated form on the skin can cause irritation.)

Spearmint. This refreshing aromatic has cleansing, calming, antiseptic, antispasmodic, decongestant and stimulating action.

Used in skin care products to help heal acne and dermatitis, spearmint also revs up the metabolism; is useful in cases of catarrh, asthma and bronchitis; acts as a soothing stomachic and digestive, and can treat nausea and vomiting.

Tangerine. Acts as a digestive, stimulant, antispasmodic, and on the lymphatic system.

Use to treat digestive disorders, obesity, nervousness and shock.

Tea-Tree. This plant gets everyone's vote for allround usefulness and effectiveness in treating the skin and fighting fungal infections and infectious disease.

Acts as an antiseptic in many skin conditions, including abscess, rashes, pruritis, dandruff, acne and herpes lesions. Fights athlete's foot and ringworm, *Candida* infections, vaginitis and infected wounds and bedsores.

Thyme. There are several varieties of thyme used by aromatherapists. They act as antibiotics, cytophylactics, antiseptics and in general are stimulating tonics for many body systems.

The individual oils are used to treat burns,

wounds and abscess; against infectious disease; to treat insomnia, anemia and asthmatic conditions.

(Caution: Some varieties of thyme will cause skin irritation if not sufficiently diluted and should not be used neat.)

Vetiver. Acts as a stimulant and a rubefacient. Used to treat arthritis and as a comforting agent for troubled psyches.

Ylang-ylang. This exotic oil has been used since ancient times to treat a variety of ailments, including baldness, oily skin and seborrhea, hypertension, heart palpitations and irregular heartbeat.

Use to promote hair growth and stimulate the scalp. It also has a calming and uplifting effect on depression and cases of stress-induced insomnia.

Chapter Four

~~~~~~~~~~~~~~~~~~~~~~~~~~~~~~

Aromatic Baths

Showers Are to Get Clean . . . Baths Make You Feel Like a Million

Before anyone thought of taking showers, there was the art and science of bathing. Bathing has always been popular whether for enjoyment, hygiene or health.

When bathing with water was considered dangerous or unfashionable, aromatics were used to cleanse and perfume the body. When bathing was in fashion, aromatics were either used as bath oil in the bath or as scented massage after the bath. In either case they acted as antiseptics and as scents, improving the hygienic value of the bath and removing personal body odors.

In ancient Egypt, those who could afford it made bathing a ritual. The first bath was cold, the second lukewarm, and the third was hot.

The hot bath was scented with aromatic oils and followed by an aromatic massage. Then the ladies had their hair dressed, their faces massaged, their breasts made up . . . No wonder Marc Antony didn't have a chance!

Not to be outdone, the ancient Syrians had private and public baths. During the greatest popularity of bathing, the king of Syria was named Antiochos. The story is told that he was once bathing in the public baths surrounded by his slaves when he was approached by a commoner. The commoner, after bowing, said how much he admired the king's aroma. The king, delighted by this show of his subject's approval, ordered a thick ointment of his perfume to be poured over the head of his admirer. This was actually a nasty idea because the recipient of the royal largesse could hardly breathe, but the king got his comeuppance. He laughed so much he slipped on the greasy ointment and landed on his behind.

Thereafter, the story goes, the king bathed in private and kept his perfume to himself.

The Greeks adopted some of the Egyptian system of aromatic bathing but not as much as the Romans did. The Greek male usually bathed in a basin in a public place and wasn't too concerned with perfumery. Greek women bathed at home.

The Romans took to bathing like a duck takes to water. Their public baths were frequented mostly by males and were an important feature of their social life. The principal baths were magnificent structures erected by the emperors. At one time there were one thousand public baths in Rome, the most magnificent being built by the Emperor Caracalla in the third century A.D.

The finest baths had a bathing ritual. On entering, you undressed first then entered a chamber called the *unctuarium* which had an assortment of perfumes and fragrant ointments. You received a preliminary scenting and then went to the cold bath or *frigidarium* for a quick dip and rubdown. Then came the *tepidarium* or tepid bath, and then the *caldarium*, the hot bath which was heated by a furnace underneath.

While in the hot bath, you scrubbed yourself all over with a *strigil*, a kind of bronze curry-comb, pouring scented oil all over you at the same time. After the bath came a relaxing massage with more fragrant oils. Those who could afford it were attended by their own slaves or by bath attendants. And this was just for the men!

The women had their baths at home, known as *cosmetae*, overseen by the ornatris, the mistress of the toilet. After the bath, the hair was styled, dyed and treated with fragrant oils. The face was massaged, the cheeks painted with *fucus*, a kind of rouge, and the eyes were shaded. Finally, the neck and shoulders were massaged with scented oils and the rest of the body lightly washed with rose water. (Sort of like a Roman version of an Elizabeth Arden salon in every household that could afford it.)

When the Roman Empire collapsed, so did bathing in Europe. People wore honey rings to keep their fleas from jumping on the table or to others. It was not until the 13th century that public bathing was reestablished, brought back by the returning crusaders. Still, bathing was not really re-established until the 17th century and it took another 200 years before Europeans were finally convinced that it was necessary and healthy to wash all over.

Of course, it was more pleasant to bathe in warm climates than in cold or chilly climes and the Europeans were afraid that bathing brought on colds and pneumonia.

Meanwhile, the Turks had observed and adopted some of the Roman bath practices and Turkish baths began to spring up. With them came the practice of using scented oils and essences again. Due to fresh memories of the Great Plague, the antiseptic powers of aromatic oils gained new respect and the scented bath became more popular than the unscented one.

The growth of the perfumed toiletries industry during the 19th and the 20th centuries has helped make bathing more of a pleasure, and now the "new" science of aromatherapy is adding new dimensions to the bathing ritual.

Aromatic baths affect us in a variety of ways. It begins with the aroma of the essences used. As it pleases the nose it pleases the soul. Then there is the physiological action of the essence on the nervous system and the rest of the body. This happens as minute amounts of the essential oils penetrate the skin, aided by the warmth and softening effect of the water, and are circulated throughout the body.

When the water is tepid the result is sedative and relaxing. When hot water is used, a short dip is tonifying but a long soak is debilitating.

So a lavender bath in tepid water is relaxing. But, if the water is too hot it will not give you the desired result. As a general rule, you know if you want to be stimulated or relaxed and will adjust the essences used and the water temperature.

There are two types of bath oils, those that dissolve in water and those that don't.

When using the oils that do not dissolve, let water into the tub, put in a few drops of the essence or essences, swish the water rather rapidly to disperse the oil and get in the tub.

Some essences are stronger than others and some people have more sensitive skin than others, so use the following sparingly: basil, pepper, peppermint, rosemary.

Use two or three drops at first, then you can increase the amount to five or six if there is no irritation. Some oils, particularly when used in combination, will add up to 12 to 15 drops collectively. You'll soon become expert in what's best for you and in what amounts.

If your skin is particularly dry, mix the essences with some of the carrier oil, put the water in the tub, add the mixture, swish the water and get in.

The bath oil which dissolves in water is usually a manufactured product of an essence and a foaming agent. It can be effective and enjoyable.

When you step out of the tub some oil will cling to the body. Towel drying will not remove all of the essence so your skin will remain lightly scented.

If you like, you can give yourself a light massage at this time or have someone else massage your body. You will be most receptive to an aromatic massage.

The combination of bathing, aromatica and massage must rank among the most relaxing luxuries a person can indulge in and one that is also good for you.

Although public bathing has now gone the way of the Dodo and showers are installed in all homes, there is no reason you cannot break the mold and help yourself by turning your tub into a spa. The sauna, on the other hand, which has become so popular in the U.S. after becoming a way of life in Finland, does not lend itself to aromatics. The purpose of the sauna is to cleanse the body through the pores. The introduction of aromatic oils via massage would have to wait for at least a half hour after the sauna session ends because the body keeps on perspiring for that long. However, if you put aside the time for a thorough cleansing, the way the Romans did, use your sauna, wait the prescribed time and then have an aromatic massage, you will find the time well spent and the results most enjoyable.

Here are a number of bath recipes you can try at home.

Invigorating Bath ~~~~~~~

To stimulate circulation and help ward off colds

3 drops juniper

2 drops peppermint

5 drops lavender

Summer Splash ～～～～

For a cooling, refreshing bath in hot weather

3 drops peppermint
4 drops bergamot
2 drops basil

Morning Energizer ～～～～

5 drops rosemary
5 drops juniper
2 drops peppermint

Sleepy-Time Soak ～～～～

2 crops chamomile
5 drops lavender
2 drops orange blossom

An Aphrodisiac Bath ～～～～

2 drops ylang-ylang
8 drops sandalwood
2 drops jasmine

Lemon-Aid to Refresh and Relax You. ～～～～

juice of ½ lemon
5 drops lemon
2 drops geranium

Note: If your skin is dry, use some carrier oil along with the essences.

Hangover Helper 〰〰〰〰

5 drops fennel
4 drops juniper
2 drops rosemary

*You can also use this combination to
make a compress for your head and to
apply in the area of the liver.*

The following list shows those oils which
are considered to be relaxing and those
considered stimulating. Use one or more according to your mood, in the amounts
suggested.

Relaxing

chamomile	2 drops
cypress	5 drops
orange blossom	2 drops
lavender	6 drops
marjoram	4 drops
rose	2 drops
sandalwood	8 drops
clary sage	4 drops

Stimulating

basil	3 drops
cardamom	4 drops
peppermint	4 drops
juniper	5 drops
hyssop	3 drops
rosemary	5 drops

Refreshing

cypress	5 drops
lemon	4 drops
peppermint	4 drops
bergamot	3 drops
geranium	4 drops
lavender	6 drops
juniper	5 drops

Aphrodisiac

jasmine	2 drops
orange blossom	2 drops
rose	2 drops
sandalwood	8 drops
ylang-ylang	3 drops

Chapter Five

Hands-On Aromatherapy

The Medium Is the Massage

Rubbing someone the wrong way, skin against skin, without the presence of a lubricant, can generate too much heat and too much pain. That is not the purpose of a massage.

Aromatherapy and massage fit like hand and glove. Using essential oils in an aromatic massage can be very beneficial. First, the selected oil or oils can penetrate the skin and second, there is the psychological effect of the massage itself and its accompanying aroma.

Massage is enjoyable to the massager and the massagee. It is a logical extension from the desire to touch a painful part of the body, to "make nice" and help relieve the stress and tension that fills our lives.

Massage is an ancient art and the terms massage and anoint mean the same thing in old texts, including the Bible. In ancient rites, oil was always present and, in most cases, scented.

Massage provides a convenient patient-healer or person-person contact. It was one of the earliest forms of healing and certainly a direct form of communication.

The hand-healer communicates healing power even when his hands are not in direct contact with the body. All of us have some healing power. We can talk with our hands and communicate what we are feeling to another being.

For this reason, you should not massage

any person if you are angry, overtired or stressed out. Your inner mood should be calm and confident.

Initially your hands may transmit a diagnosis to you of the massagee. You'll notice tension in the muscles, painful spots, swollen areas and old sprains and strains. Then, while still diagnosing, your hands will begin to transmit the healing power of the aromatic essences and the power of two people in harmony.

It is a good idea to get a massage from an expert before you attempt to give a massage. Until then, gentle massaging with the essences will permit the aromatics to do their thing and keep you from doing any damage with deep, neuromuscular massage movements.

Your massage has three aims:

- To aid the penetration of the essence through the skin
- To either stimulate or relax the individual
- To treat a condition locally

For most effective penetration of the therapeutic oils, the skin must be clean and free of other oils or lotions.

Of course, massage therapists are the experts at this, but anyone can learn to give a simple, soothing massage to a loved one or friend. There are several things to keep in mind to make the experience as relaxing and enjoyable as possible:

• Make sure the environment is conducive to relaxation. Turn off the phone or lock the doors to guard against interruptions. Quiet, instrumental music is nice. The room should feel slightly warm to the masseur or masseuse.

• Select a carrier oil and an essence for the mood or result you wish to achieve, or have the person select one he or she likes.

• Warm the oil slightly if possible.

• Try and keep an unbroken flow to your strokes, with one hand on the person at all times to avoid sudden stops and starts.

• Always pour the oil into your hands before rubbing it on the person, and use only as much as you need at a time. You can always apply more.

• Take your cues from the person being massaged. Only talk if he or she seems to want to. Otherwise, enjoy the silence.

Swedish Massage. Swedish massage is most familiar to people. One of the typical movements is called *effleurage*. It starts with long, slow, gentle strokes of the entire hand over the back and the rest of the body. The strokes are always made in the direction of the heart.

Kneading movements are next. These warm up the muscles for deeper work, which includes hacking and pounding movements. These have their therapeutic uses but are not for amateurs to tackle.

Reflexology. Reflexology is another form of hands-on healing which can be done in conjunction with aromatherapy. Reflexologists work on the foot, stroking the entire foot and then concentrating on an area that corresponds to the part of the person's body that might need extra help.

Often called zone therapy, it is more than a massage. Reflexology is also a diagnostic and a treatment tool when used by a competent reflexologist. Although there are reflex points throughout the body, for our purposes here we will consider only the feet, which are the focal point of a reflexology massage.

Zone therapy operates on the principle that there are ten zones in the human body, with half of the zones on each side of a vertical, central line. All of the organs that are in the middle part of our bodies are encompassed in the first zone of both feet. Certain organs found only in one part of the body are in the zone of the corresponding foot. For example, the spleen is on the left side of the body, so to treat the spleen you refer to the left foot.

A basic tenet of reflexology is, "If it hurts, massage it." Reflexology massage is done with the side of the thumb, moving in small circles. Any pain, called a reflex pain, won't be felt as a typical foot pain. Instead, the subject may jump or flinch. This means there is very likely a problem in the corresponding area of the body.

You can't harm yourself or anyone else by

trying reflexology, as long as you do it gently and without exerting too much pressure. Aromatherapy is well-suited to reflexology massage because the surface area of the foot absorbs the essential oil easily.

Shiatsu. Shiatsu is another type of fairly vigorous massage, which is a type of oriental medicine. The translation from the Japanese is literally "finger pressure." It is not a deep muscle massage; rather, the energy points of the body, called meridians, are lightly massaged to release the energy and life force of the body.

Again, for nonprofessionals, a soothing more superficial massage is probably the best to try. Always lighten up if your subject shows signs of pain in a particular area or tenses up.

If there is a particular problem, such as an aching ankle or shoulder, the massage can be aimed at that area, but for a full body massage it's best to start with the back, hands or feet so the other party is already relaxed when you begin to attend to the rest of the body.

Have your subject avoid showering for about six hours after a massage with essential oils, to take full advantage of the penetrating powers of the essences and oils. Refer to the first chapter for tips on mixing your own massage blends.

Karin Burling is a registered massage therapist in Houston, Texas who only began using aromatherapy in her practice after being certified a year ago. She finds it fascinating that even her most skeptical clients find aromatherapy treatment "very effective" once they give it a try.

She has a number of pregnant clients that have responded well to the combination of massage and essential oils: "One client who was eight months pregnant had the typical build-up of fluid, particularly in her lower legs," Karin recalls. Using gentle massage with a blend of citrus oils, rosewood and tangerine, Karin was able to significantly reduce the edema and make the woman more comfortable. Plus, the beneficial effects were long-lasting.

Lower back pain is a problem for many, but especially women. "I work with many people who suffer from lower back pain," says Karin, "and I find that juniper is consistently helpful for this nagging problem."

Penny Zenglein of San Luis Obispo, California started out as an aerobics instructor and became interested in the therapeutic aspects of massage therapy after watching her mother, who practices in Washington. Now a licensed massage therapist herself, she incorporates many aspects of aromatherapy into her work.

Zenglein has taken several aromatherapy courses, including studying under Dr. Daniel Penoel of France, who with his wife Rosemary now runs a health clinic in England and teaches aromatherapy around the world.

She also enjoys experimenting with the many properties of the essential oils herself. She says certain formulas definitely help stimulate memory, and that she "aced a test" after using a little rosemary and ginger root to aid her concentration.

Most of her clients come to her for stress reduction, and although she notes she cannot prescribe essential oils of course, she helps clients who indicate they are open to the potential of aromatherapy select a massage oil or scent to match any symptoms they may be experiencing.

"Tension headaches respond almost immediately to a dot of peppermint on the temples," she explains, "and a neck and shoulder massage with a lavender blend can reduce muscle tension and aches in that area for days." For someone who needs a quick picker-upper, "rosemary and peppermint act as a stimulating, overall tonic."

Her favorite essential oils are tea-tree ("put a dab on a cotton swab and apply to a canker sore for fast relief"), lavender, peppermint, eucalyptus and rosemary.

Therapeutic Massage Mixtures

Massages can be helpful or sensual or both. Sensual massage needs no explanation so we'll concentrate on helpful massages.

Muscle aches are usually caused by a build-up of lactic acid. By massaging the muscle groups, starting off with a very gentle pressure and gradually building up pressure almost to the point of pain, the lactic acid can be dispersed as more blood is brought to the affected tissues. Remember to massage in a circular motion, and always upwards toward the heart, never toward the feet.

Aching Arms ~~~~~~~~~~

7 drops lavender
7 drops rosemary
8 drops juniper
to 50 cc vegetable oil

Aching Legs ~~~~~~~~~~

15 drops lavender
10 drops rosemary
to 50 cc vegetable oil

For Menstrual Cramps ~~~~~~~

12 drops clary sage
to 50 cc vegetable oil

It took only two sessions of massage combined with aromatherapy for Tara Kamath to become hooked. Tara, a licensed massage therapist who works in the Santa Monica area and lives in Malibu, was being massaged by her former instructor during the first part of her period, when she usually experiences painful cramps. He offered to use essential oils on her in conjunction with the massage, oils blended specifically to help the painful muscle contractions.

After the second massage a month later, at the same time during her cycle, Tara realized her dreaded cramps had disappeared completely. Tara wanted to learn all about this new therapy herself—and now teaches aromatherapy to other massage practitioners in southern California, along with using it regularly in her private practice.

"Aromatherapy is a wonderful tool everybody can use at least to some extent themselves," she explains. "As soon as I started to use it, I really felt an affinity with it." Along the way, she studied Oriental medicine, and Chinese herbal medicine. Now she continues her studies into the chemistry of aromatherapy's effect on the body.

"I learned a lot about the plants through my herbal studies, and certainly having that basic understanding of the plant world has helped me. But the essential oils of a plant do not necessarily have the same properties as herbs derived from the same plant, so my studies in aromatherapy seemed a logical progression for me."

Breast-Enlarging Massage Oil ~

Although there are no guarantees, many people have been delighted with this massage mixture:

10 drops geranium oil.
12 drops ylang-ylang oil
to 50 cc vegetable oil

Massage morning and evening but do not overdo it.

To Trim Thighs 〜〜〜〜〜

10 drops juniper
10 drops cypress
to 50 cc vegetable oil

In the Mood 〜〜〜〜〜〜

(An aphrodisiac massage oil)
Mix:
6 drops rose oil
4 drops jasmine
4 drops bergamot
8 drops sandalwood
to 50 cc vegetable oil

Begin by massaging yourself until the aroma attracts him. Then begin to massage him and let him massage you. It's really a magical mixture!

Wake-up Massage 〜〜〜〜〜

2 drops geranium
5 drops orange
15 drops rosewood
to 50 cc vegetable oil

This is a refreshing mixture which stimulates the circulation and will get you on your feet and into exercising.

Relaxing Massage 〜〜〜〜〜〜

Just the opposite . . . for winding down!
8 drops sandalwood
2 drops geranium
10 drops lavender
to 50 cc vegetable oil

To Treat Stretch Marks ～～～

These unsightly marks can come from giving birth and from heavy exercise as well
as from gaining and losing weight. Massage gently every other day with:

15 drops lavender
5 drops neroli
to 50 cc vegetable oil

Chapter Six

Creating an Aromatic Environment

The use of aromatic fumigations is probably as old as humanity. Priests, sorcerers, healers of all traditions used them extensively in their ceremonies and various rituals. Ancient Egyptians burned perfumes in the streets and inside the temples. More than 2,000 years ago, Hippocrates, the father of Western medicine, successfully struggled against the epidemic of plague in Athens, using aromatic fumigations throughout the city. In the Middle Ages, people burned pine or other fragrant woods in the streets in time of epidemic to cast out the devils. Perfumers were often worn around the neck to help the wearer resist diseases.

Nowadays, there is a new smokeless process. Coming from Europe where it is quite popular in the natural therapy movement, the aromatic diffuser is an apparatus that diffuses essential oils in the air without altering or heating them. The ionized microparticles, which stay suspended for several hours, revitalize the air by their antiseptic and deodorant action. The oxidation of the essential oils causes low doses of natural ozone to decompose in oxygen ions. This process, which occurs naturally in forests, has an invigorating and purifying effect.

The aromatic diffuser projects drops of essential oils in a Pyrex nebulizer, using air as a propellant. The nebulizer acts as an expansion chamber where the drops of oil are broken into a very thin mist. Since air is the gas propellant, there is no chemical pollution, no alteration of the oils or decomposition by heat.

There has been a lot of clinical research on the use of this apparatus over the last ten years. A thinner diffusion gives better results. Then, besides the antiseptic action already widely documented, there is a very strong action on the lungs and the respiratory system in general (useful for treating asthma, bronchitis, colds, sinusitis, sore throats, etc.). The action on the circulatory system, the heart and the nervous system is also very pronounced.

In fact, the aromatic diffuser can be used for almost all the prescriptions of aromatherapy. It is the subtlest, easiest and most pleasant way to take essential oils. In France, many naturopathic and yoga centers use this apparatus. It can be installed in any public or private place where air treatment is needed: saunas, hot tubs, hospitals, consulting rooms, waiting rooms, gymnastic centers, schools and of course at home, in any room.

There is an obvious connection between the psychic centers and the lungs. Most spiritual practices emphasize the importance of breathing. The aromatic diffuser, then, is the best way to experience the subtle effects of essential oils on the spirit and the soul. By contributing to the creation of a cheerful atmosphere, it enhances the quality of life, giving it a taste of natural elegance. It is thus a precious tool for the holistic practitioner.

Suggested Oils

The sense of smell is very subjective; you might particularly like some fragrances and dislike some others. Plus, your appreciation will vary, depending on your mood, the time of the day, the season. But here are some general suggestions on using essential oils in your own diffuser.

- Calming (evening): lavender, marjoram, chamomile
- Stimulant (morning): sage, rosemary, pine, mints
- Aphrodisiac: ylang-ylang, sandalwood, ginger, peppermint, pepper, savory
- For the lungs: eucalyptus, lavender, pine, cajuput, copaiba, hyssop
- For nervousness: mugwort, petitgrain, marjoram, neroli
- Against hypertension: ylang-ylang, lavender, lemon, marjoram
- Against hypotension: hyssop, sage, thyme, rosemary
- Antidepressants: frankincense, myrrh, cedarwood
- Purifiers: lavandin, lemon grass, lemon, pine, chamomile, geranium, oregano
- Revivifiers: pine, fir, black spruce
- To strengthen the brain and fortify memory: basil, juniper, rosemary
- To treat insomnia: neroli, marjoram, chamomile

When you first step into the aromatic world of essential oils, you might be a little bit surprised, or even slightly turned off. Your olfactory system may have to be reeducated, or rather, detoxified. After years of neglect and abuse with junk perfumes, your nose might not be able to fully appreciate the richness of natural fragrances. When you change your eating habits from junk food to a more healthy diet, you cannot really appreciate the full flavor of a lettuce leaf, a plain radish or a bowl of brown rice at first. But after you start to detoxify, your taste greatly improves and refines. Soon you do not want to come back to junk again. In this manner the power of fragrances is revealed to you every day as you play with them, dance with them, create with them. They connect you to the quintessence of the realm of plants and will "make thee glad, merry, gracious and well-beloved of all men."

Chapter Seven

Towards a More Beautiful You

Aromatics have a tradition of use in skin care which goes back some 5,000 years and maybe further. The ancient Egyptians were probably the first to use aromatic toiletries to any extent. They prepared scented oils, unguents, and facial masks. Modern women would turn down a line of Egyptian cosmetics because they were too heavy and sticky, but the Egyptians treasured their early adventures into this area.

Just as modern medicine has become oriented to the test tube and the laboratory, so have modern cosmetics. Products have become synthetic and unnatural and people react badly to many of the ingredients. It would be good for us if we could find natural answers to our cosmetic problems.

Essential oils are an ideal form in which to use plants for skin care because they lend themselves to mixing with creams, lotions, ointments, perfumes and so on. When taking a facial, the scent is as important as the entire practice. The scents help you relax, which is important to the practical end of the facial. Relaxed muscles respond more readily to treatment than those which are tense or in spasm.

Floral Essences

The flower oils such as jasmine, rose, ylang-ylang, neroli and chamomile seem to be the most useful in this area and the most popular.

The theme of French biochemist Marguerite Maury's book, *The Secret of Life and Youth*, is rejuvenation and she suggests that essential oils are natural rejuvenating agents and form a viable alternative to other methods.

Those other methods usually involve some type of treatment with animal extracts (including hormones, placenta or cellular extracts). How can the products of death bring rejuvenation?

According to Maury's book, "Applied to the skin these essences regulate the activity of the capillaries and restore vitality to the tissues. We might almost say that they make the flesh more succulent."

Facialist and massage therapist Linda-Ann Kahn turned a busy private "aesthetic" aromatherapy practice into an aromatherapy day spa that has been thriving for nine years now. Kahn and her staff of 23 at the Beauty Kliniek in San Diego work with essential oils every day, particularly in the 10 different treatments offered at the luxurious salon.

Kahn was first introduced to aromatherapy in her native South Africa, back in 1978, and began studying it extensively in 1983 when she realized the tremendous benefits—both personally and for her clientele. Always looking to expand her knowledge, Kahn has since incorporated acupressure, hydrotherapy, visualization and reflexology into her protocol, feeling that all these facets of her work enhance each other.

"I custom blend the facial or body oils according to what's going on for that person, physically, emotionally, psychologically," she explains.

She has had success in treating skin problems from acne to eczema using aromatherapy in cosmetology treatments. "For eczema, I may use bergamot, juniper, blue camomile, and then whatever else the person may need, whether it's something to help calm them or lift their spirits.

"To treat acne, I use apricot kernel oil as a carrier oil. Almond is heavier so you never use that on that type of skin. To the base oil I add juniper, bergamot which is very disinfecting, roman chamomile, maybe carrotseed oil. In severe acne where the lymph system is affected, I use rosemary, which acts on that system and helps promote drainage."

For someone who is feeling down or depressed, Linda may use clary sage in the diffuser during a massage or beauty treatment, because this essential oil is uplifting, while others who need an energy boost or calming influence require something else.

A nice warm, bubbling whirlpool is a wonderful way to relax, but at the Kliniek it becomes European-style hydrotherapy with 77 jets of water gently massaging you. And, according to your desired mood, essential oils can be added to the tub to help stimulate your energy, or an anti-stress mixture can help soothe away a bad week at work.

Another treatment at the day spa that shows the surprising power of aromatherapy is a body wrap. "After a client gets out of the tub, we wrap her in a cold, wet sheet which has essential oils in it. Women are always amazed that they don't feel cold. The oils in the wrap warm you, and help draw your energy into the center."

You can even treat your tootsies to a predicure with essential oils, or purchase the salon's synthetic-free perfumes.

It is possible to improve one's general health—including the health and appearance of the skin—through natural health care and skin care. This improvement includes diet, exercise, supplements, good sleep habits, drinking lots of water and avoidance of cigarettes and alcohol.

Apart from the general process of improving health, essential oils also increase the elimination of waste matter and dead cells and contribute to the growth of new, healthy cells. Reminiscent of the ancient Egyptians and their ability to preserve flesh by embalming, certain essences are antiseptic in nature. Not only are they able to ward off the attacks of bacteria, but they also prevent the growth of most fungi. The regular use of essential oils and aromatic skin care is the safest and surest way to achieve a healthy, rejuvenated complexion.

For older individuals, the use of the heavier essences such as frankincense, sandalwood and myrrh, seems to yield the best results. We have seen mature people with the skin of a 20-year-old—not often but once in a while—and lighter essences are then recommended in these cases.

A number of factors can cause the skin to age prematurely. Some we can control, while other factors are beyond our control.

We cannot control the garbage in the air, the harsh environment that beats at the skin with dirt, pollutants, harmful rays from the sun and so on. Then there's the drying of the skin and the loss of elasticity, which yields wrinkles and flabby skin. Add in blackheads, poor pallor, pimples . . .

Not a pretty thought and even less a pretty sight! But all is not lost.

Most essences are *cytophylactic*, that is, they stimulate the generation of new cells. This ability helps preserve the health and youth of the skin and, in many cases, can actually restore the appearance of youth.

This cytophylactic property is particularly evident in oils of lavender and orange blossom. This is one reason that lavender is so good for healing burns.

However, it is not necessary to use these essences in every preparation since all essences share this ability to some degree. You may like one essence better than the other because you react better to it.

Millions of dollars have been spent on hormone creams because they have the reputation for rejuvenating the skin. In aromatherapy, fennel oil, which contains estrogens, has a reputation as an anti-wrinkle cream. Other essences contain phytohormones (plant hormones) or have a hormonal action which benefits both dry and oily skin, provokes a firming effect on the skin, stimulates the metabolism of the skin cells, and collectively, exert a rejuvenating action.

Essential oils are natural, organic substances which work in harmony with the natural forces of the body. *You* have to help. You can't smoke and be rejuvenated. Nor can you abuse your digestive system and be rejuvenated. The look of your skin reflects the state of your body, which in turn reflects the state of your mind and your lifestyle. The health of the skin depends strongly on the blood. The blood is only as nourishing as the food you eat and the supplements you take in support of your diet. Metabolic waste products can build up in the tissues causing congestion and, because the skin is one of the waste-removal organs in the body, it will reflect this underlying condition of *dis-ease* or poor health.

Most essential oils should not be used without being diluted since they can be irritating to sensitive skin. Some, such as mustard or wintergreen, are highly irritating, while others such as eucalyptus and camphor are mildly irritating. Therefore, almost all formulas call for combinations of the essences with carrier oils or dilutions with water or alcohol.

Some aromatherapists stress the need for deodorized alcohol, but that is almost impossible to obtain. Grain alcohol is the best to use but you need a special license to buy it.

I recommend a good bottle of vodka. It is odorless, inexpensive and does the job.

Cosmetic Formulas

Dry Skin Oil ~~~~~~~~~
5 drops sandalwood
5 drops geranium
3 drops rosewood
4 drops ylang-ylang
in 2 ounces carrier oil

Acne. Diet and supplements are important to the treatment of this condition, including vitamins, garlic capsules, G.L.A., zinc and other minerals. Avoid iodine-containing foods.

Try a facial steam with lavender, bergamot and geranium twice a week. Use wheat germ and/or avocado oil as the carrier oil when you make up your massage treatment. Use the massage oil gently once a week.

Aromatic baths regularly with rosemary, cypress, chamomile, juniper and sandalwood.

An Acne Formula ~~~~~~~~
10 drops cypress
11 drops lemon
in 2 ounces carrier oil

Gentle massage once a week.

Massage Oil for Mature Skin ~~
8 drops frankincense
13 drops of lavender
2 drops neroli
in 2 ounces carrier oil

Facial Oil for Inflamed Skin ⌇

Chamomile is very soothing

5 drops chamomile
3 drops neroli
2 drops rose
in 2 ounces carrier oil

For Oily Skin ⌇

8 drops bergamot
3 drops cypress
4 drops juniper
in 2 ounces carrier oil

Oily skin will also respond to the use of the following mixture:

6 drops tea-tree
9 drops cypress
5 drops lemon
5 drops geranium
in 2 ounces grapeseed oil as a carrier.

The same mixture can be used as a compress.

Greasy Skin ⌇

6 drops bergamot
2 drops lavender
in 2 ounces carrier oil

Tonic Waters for Your Complexion ⌇

4 drops bergamot
10 drops jasmine
in 2 ounces distilled water

4 drops geranium (for dry skin only)
6 drops lavender
in 2 ounces distilled water

7 drops rose
10 drops bergamot
in 2 ounces distilled water

7 drops cypress
10 drops juniper
in 2 ounces distilled water

6 drops lavender (for oily skin only)
10 drops bergamot
in 2 ounces distilled water

You can use bottled spring water instead of distilled water if you wish.

For Alopecia (Baldness) ～～～

10 drops juniper
7 drops lavender
7 drops rosemary
in 2 ounces carrier oil.

Massage into scalp and leave on for one hour. Apply shampoo to hair and rub in before adding water. This will make the mixture easy to remove.

Dandruff or Oily Hair 〰〰〰

7 drops cedarwood
10 drops cypress
10 drops juniper
in 2 ounces carrier oil

Massage into the scalp and leave on for one hour. Add shampoo and work in well before lathering with water. This makes the mix easy to remove.

Facial Mask 〰〰〰〰〰〰

Make a mixture of
1 heaping tablespoon fuller's earth or kaolin
2 tablespoons water
½ teaspoon honey
1 drop lavender
1 drop geranium

Masks are for deep cleansing. They can be made from fuller's earth or kaolin (available at a health store), like the above, plus items such as yogurt, fruit and essences.

Yogurt is cleansing, toning, extractive and mild enough for all skin types. Always use live yogurt because its activity depends on the bacteria it contains. It must be mixed with kaolin or fuller's earth because it is too slippery alone.

Dry skin needs a mild moisturizing mask. Fruit is ideal for this purpose. Peel the fruit and pulp it, add a bit of honey, the base material of kaolin and a drop or two of the essential oil. You can add a bit of wheat germ oil for dry, mature skin.

Oily skin responds well to additional brewer's yeast in the basic mix to help remove impurities.

Mask Formulas

Acne—*cabbage, grape, tomato, yeast, camphor, juniper, bergamot*

Oily skin—cabbage, grape, lemon, pear, strawberry, camphor, frankincense

Sensitive skin—honey and yogurt, grape, melon, neroli, rose, chamomile

Dry skin—avocado, banana, carrot, melon, wheat germ oil, rose, sandalwood.

Mature skin—apple, avocado, grape, lemon, wheat germ oil, cypress, frankincense, patchouli

Normal skin—avocado, grape, lemon, peach, wheat germ oil, jasmine, neroli, lavender

Use one or two ingredients in each list and one or two essences. The mask stimulates circulation, promotes the elimination of waste material and nourishes the skin.

Use a facial mask every one or two weeks, leave on for up to 20 minutes, then gently sponge off with warm water. Tissue-dry the skin by patting gently.

Of course, not all of us have the time or wherewithal to concoct our own aromatherapy preparations. A look around your favorite health store, however, will reveal a treasure trove of products.

There are:

• Herbal facial steams. Tea bags filled with a combination of herbs and essential oils designed for acne, oily or dry skin or for sensitive skin use.

• Herbal mitts. Soap, herbs and essential oils in a glove you can rub over your body in the shower. Some of the combinations are designed to wake you up while others help you to relax for sleep.

If you have trouble remembering your dreams, there's even a pad of scented violet to place under your pillow.

• Beauty grains. Just mix with yogurt and honey to make a facial mask for deep cleansing and a velvet skin.

• Bath beads. Essential oils and vitamin E for your bath.

• Skin and lip protectants. Moisturizing protection from the damaging rays of the sun with flower and plant essences.

• Scalp and hair care products for normal, oily or dry scalps.

And lots, lots more. Ask about aromatherapeutic products at your health food store or herbal practitioner's.

Chapter Eight

~~~~~~~~~~~~~~~~~~~~~~~~~~~~~~~~~~~~~

Using Scents to
Stir the Psyche

Psychosomatic, meaning having components that are both mental and physical, refers to a condition that is emotional in origin but physical in manifestation. It used to be used in a derisive manner, mostly as a tool against women. However, the medical profession is now beginning to understand that it cannot separate the physical and mental when considering therapy. Physical conditions such as asthma and colitis, for example, are often considered to have strong psychosomatic elements.

The fact that our mental condition has a strong bearing on our physical condition should not be surprising. We are one entity. Yet we cannot consider mind and body to be identical. The body remains after death but the mind does not go with it to the grave. However, the two do interact, each affecting the other.

The mind affects the body primarily through the autonomic nervous system, and can overstimulate the glands that are controlled by that system. For example, if the mind stimulates an oversecretion of gastric juice containing hydrochloric acid, it can cause an ulcer over a period of time. Many digestive disorders may be mind-triggered, especially cramps and constipation.

Bach Flower Remedies

Dr. Edward Bach, a physician of great insight who originated the Bach Flower Remedies, said it was the duty of the physician to administer such remedies as will help the physical body to gain strength and assist the mind to become calm, widen its outlook and strive toward perfection, thus bringing peace and harmony to the whole personality.

The Bach flower remedies are, like aromatherapy, another form of phytotherapy (*phyto* meaning plant). You may wish to consider these remedies as an adjunct to aromatherapy treatment. Dr. Bach gave up his traditional medical practice in Wales in 1930 to develop his remedies, which are prepared from the flowers of wild plants, including trees and bushes. The purpose of these 38 remedies is to affect the mental state behind the ailments.

As Bach envisioned and used them, the flower remedies improve your overall health and well-being subtly. He believed that, by creating your own harmony and finding inner peace, you could heal yourself. Whereas the essential oils used by aromatherapists affect you on a physical, mental and emotional level simultaneously, the Bach flower treatments are a form of self-help for the psyche, with an assist from Mother Nature.

There are a number of good books on this subject (including the several listed at the end of this book in the bibliography) to guide you to the proper use of these remedies. They are also a fascinating way to uncover the negative personality traits that may be affecting your health.

Furthermore, the remedies are safe and have no side effects since, if your body doesn't need the remedy you've chosen to take, it just won't use it.

Some remedies, such as walnut, may be called for only in periods of stress. Walnut helps you deal with change or transition, which, whether it is a good change (such as new job) or a bad change (a divorce), affects your mental health and stress level the same. Holly can be used to treat jealousy, for another example, while crab apple can release you from nagging thoughts of despair or a general feeling of despondency. Crab apple also helps people who have trouble keeping things in perspective. These are just a few examples of Bach's remedies, which have a proven record since he developed them decades ago.

Essences can be of use as therapeutic agents in the same way that many chemicals are now used, except the essences work in a more subtle, natural way without the characteristic side effects of many synthetic chemicals.

Consider that aromatics, such as incense, were used first as calming agents to induce a state of contentment. Sounds like one of our modern-day tranquilizers, however the aromatic—unlike the pills—is completely safe.

In general, essences have an uplifting quality and, at the same time, a calming virtue. As far back as ancient Greece, the physician Galen recommended the use of aromatic herbs against hysterical convulsions. Burning bay leaves were inhaled by the Oracle at Delphi to induce a trancelike state enabling communication with the gods. Aromatic woods were later burned to drive out "evil spirits." Even then, aroma was known to have an effect on the psyche.

Dwight Hines, Ph.D. explained in the *Journal of Altered States of Consciousness* (Vol. 3(1):17–39, 1977) that odors are capable of creating "an emotional, ecstatic state of consciousness that would render individuals more susceptible to religious experience," which may account in part for the importance of incense and odor in religious ceremonies and rituals.

This is not to say that essences are curealls. They are very useful crutches against some depressive states but they cannot solve the underlying situation which induced the state originally.

I must make this point because I don't want anyone to sniff ylang-ylang and ignore medical treatment if it is warranted.

Professor Giovanni Rovesti in his book *In Search of Perfumes Lost* tells of studying the effects of essences on the psyche. He comments:

> According to sociologists and neurologists, the salient characteristics of our age are those of anxiety and depression, and material proof is available in the ever higher figures shown for the comsumption of tranquilizers and stimulants. It is well known that disturbance and toxicosis can be caused by these products if taken regularly.

Both neuroses often cause aversion to any type of pleasure, by producing a sense of weariness which many people are unable to overcome.

The possibility of applying new therapies to these widespread psycho-neuroses is therefore of considerable importance.

For such purposes, therefore, interest attaches to the use of essential oils as aids, or even as sole remedies in psychotherapy.

The matter is of still further interest, since the essential oils that are employed in aromatherapy, in the appropriate doses, are harmless to the organism and do not cause troubles like those produced by ordinary psychological drugs.

Rovesti does not suggest that essences can take the place of psychotherapy in its many and varied forms, but that they form a useful and safer adjunct to such therapies than chemical tranquilizers. However, essences are not to be thought of as miracle drugs in the case of severe mental disturbance. They are only adjuncts to professional help.

Memory Stimulants

Early on in this book it was revealed that the sense of smell in the brain is closely related to the more primitive self and that the nose provides a direct passage to the brain. This means that odors do not have to pass the blood/brain barrier which has been set up by nature to block the entrance of harmful substances. Smell and touch evoke our most primitive emotions and the most likely to be loaded with instinctive reactions. It is strange that olfactory nerve cells (the cells connected to the sense of smell) can be replaced. Other nerve cells, such as those in the brain, the ear or the eye, cannot be replaced. Nature doesn't do things without a reason so this underlines the importance of the ability to smell.

Memory and smell are linked. Claims that certain oils have the ability to stimulate concentration and memory go back to antiquity. Oils with strong, piercing odors—like basil, peppermint and rosemary—are considered the most potent in this respect.

Essential oils stimulate the central nervous system, thereby increasing our ability to concentrate. This leads to an improvement in memory.

Why should this be so?

The ability to smell and the ability to remember both live in the limbic system. Not close to each other but *in the same area.*

The limbic system, or the old brain, developed some 70 million years ago. It was one of the first parts to develop. The cortex, the part of the brain which performs intellectual duties, didn't form until much later. The old name for the limbic section was *rhinencephalon*, which literally means smell-brain. This smell-brain is implicated in the emotional responses of pleasure, pain, rage, docility, anger, fear, sorrow, affection and sexual feelings.

Quite a lot to expect from so "primitive" a bunch of nerve tissue!

Animal experiments using essential oils showed that fennel or rosemary made dogs apprehensive while hyssop or sage caused them to become aggressive. Clary sage and ylang-ylang brought on a docile attitude. But of course, dogs are not people.

Massage therapist and aromatherapy instructor Tara Kamath of Malibu, California believes that several well-chosen, ready-made blends are a good place for novices to start experiencing the scent-sations of essential oils.

"This is also a safe and pleasant way to get the feel of aromatic oils and their properties. The French medical approach often relies on high doses of essential oils but laypeople should never try this.

"Besides, a smaller dose often works at least as well, and doesn't put stress on the body the way larger doses from a physician may. Also, you may need to grow accustomed to some of the smells, after abusing your nose with synthetics and petrochemicals. But after a while of retraining your nose, you'll find it's easy to tell the difference between a synthetic blend and an essential oil."

Informed clients who open up when Kamath asks them "what's going on" in their lives give her clues that enable her to select an oil that will soothe their jagged psyches, calm anxious nerves about an impending important meeting, relax them and get them in a vacation frame of mind, or act as a stimulating pick-up to rev them up for a week of work. And there are certain oils that people respond to that trigger beloved memories, perhaps of a grandparent or the home where they grew up.

Before leaving this area of aromatherapy, there is one very strange fact that we ought to know. We've been taught in school that the nerves that originate in the left part of the brain control the action of the right side of the body and vice-versa. That's entirely true for all of the senses—*except* the sense of smell.

The olfactory nerves do not cross over. The left nostril leads to the left side of the brain—the logical part. The right nostril leads to the right side of the brain—the intuitive part. The left nostril identifies odors easily while the right nostril reacts to odors emotionally.

The relationship between scent and the right brain may help explain the ability of aromatherapy to produce euphoria and a distancing from anxiety. Unlike chemical drugs, essences promote creative thoughts and pleasant feelings instead of suppressing them and, of course, the essences are non-addictive.

Part of the psychological effect of essential oils is due to the way they smell. The most universally pleasing oils, such as jasmine and rose, have the most potential for aromatherapy. Blends of essences that have particular scent appeal to an individual will have the best results for that person. (Many herbal practitioners believe this attraction toward certain scents is an instinctual action, that you will be drawn to the essences your body most needs. This parallels the Bach flower remedies, in which their effect depends solely on your individual needs.)

Of course it is not possible to define precise limits or precise action of aromatics. We are still so individual that some scents perceived as attractive to some may have unpleasant connotations to others. So, although the final reaction is up to the individual, the following table is accurate in general.

Psychological Properties of Essences

To Alleviate These Conditions	Try One or More
Anxiety and Nervous Tension	benzoin, bergamot, chamomile, cypress, geranium, jasmine, lavender, marjoram, melissa, neroli, rose, ylang-ylang
Depression	basil, bergamot, chamomile, geranium, jasmine, lavender, neroli, peppermint, rose, sandalwood, ylang-ylang

To Alleviate These Conditions	*Try One or More*
Anger	chamomile, melissa, rose, ylang-ylang
Apathy	jasmine, juniper, rosemary
Confusion	basil, cypress, frankincense, peppermint
Dwelling on the past	benzoin, frankincense
Fear or Paranoia	basil, clary sage, jasmine, juniper
Grief	hyssop, marjoram, rose
Hypersensitivity	chamomile, jasmine, melissa
Hypochondria	melissa, jasmine
Irritability	chamomile, cypress, lavender, marjoram, rose
Jealousy	rose
Panic	chamomile, clary sage, jasmine, lavender, marjoram, melissa, neroli, ylang-ylang
Shock	melissa, neroli
Suspicion	lavender

Chapter Nine

A Compendium of
Essential Oils

Care Of Your Essential Oils

Essential oils are all highly volatile which means they will readily evaporate if given half a chance. So store them in dark-colored bottles in a cool place and make sure that the stoppers are tight.

Buy your oils in small amounts and don't kick if they're expensive. If you are careful, the oils will last for up to five years, but for best results change your oils at least once a year. Orange, lemon, and grapefruit, on the other hand, last no more than six months but they are not as expensive as most of the other aromatics.

Buy natural essences. There are some un-ethical companies which try to pass off per-fumes of synthetic products under the name of fragrance oils or aromatic oils. Insist on essential oils and read the labels carefully.

The Most Commonly Used Essential Oils

Clary Sage
Salvia sclarea

Essence obtained from: herb and flowers

Odor: floral and herbaceous

Usually imported from: France

Most common uses:
   depression
   menstrual pain
   premenstrual syndrome (PMS)

This plant is related to the common sage, but the essences have different values. Since ordinary sage has been known to be toxic, it is not recommended for aromatherapy use.

Its name probably is a reflection of its early use for clearing the eyes, since a mucilage from the seed was used to remove foreign particles from the eye.

The plant has a long history of use as both a food and a medicine. The leaves were served as a vegetable after being dipped in batter and deep-fried. In Germany, wine merchants mixed it with their Rhine wine to achieve a muscatel-like flavor.

Clary sage has euphoric effect when evaporated into the air or used in a massage. It is one of the most effective elements for relieving depressive states.

This essence can also be tapped for its capacity to stimulate the sexual appetite. The musky odor of the essential oil justifies its use as a sensual massage oil. The euphoria is a link to this aphrodisiac reputation. Researchers suspect it increases the release of adrenaline and estrogen, which also makes the case for its use in treating menstrual disorders, period pain and pre-menstrual syndrome. In the case of PMS, its ability to lift the spirits is of great value.

Lavender
Lavandula officinalis

Essence obtained from: flowering tops

Odor: floral and herbaceous

Cultivated in: France, Tasmania

Most common uses:
   burns
   bites and stings
   eczema
   dermatitis
   insomnia
   nervous tension
   anxiety
   asthma
   immune deficiency (persistent infections)
   head and body lice

Lavender, in today's world, is so well-known that its name is instantly associated, not only with its fragrance, but with the distinctive mauve-like color of its tiny petals. It has been known since ancient times and was extremely popular with pre-Christian Greeks and Romans who used the oil to scent their baths and soaps. From that usage probably came its Latin name, from *lavare*, to wash, and its anglicized name, lavender.

By the Dark Ages, though, the sensuous joy of lavender condemned it to relative obscurity behind a list of other herbs used only for religious or medicinal purposes. It wasn't until the late Renaissance that the celebrated fragrance was released from obscurity along with Tudor England.

In 1694, the oil was promoted as a treatment for head lice and as a fumigant for sick rooms but that did not damage its reputation or its wonderful fragrance.

Lavender is one of the mildest yet most effective of the essential oils and should be number one on your list of oils to buy. Burns, headaches, indigestion, insect bites and stings, infections, sores, dermatitis—all these common complaints can be soothed with this magic oil. It is antiseptic, relaxing, analgesic and healing.

In the 17th and 18th centuries, ladies would drench themselves in lavender water to protect against foul smells and fainting.

Medicinally, lavender is capable of stimulating both the production and the activity of certain white blood cells, thereby stimulating the body's immune system. Lavender also appears able to stimulate cellular growth and, in that manner, contributes to rejuvenation.

Peppermint
Mentha piperita

Essence obtained from: leaves

Odor: minty

Cultivated in: United States, Brazil, Europe

Most common uses:
nausea
indigestion
colic
diarrhea
flatulence
headache

pain
mental fatigue
influenza
colds
sinus congestion

It started a long, long time ago when Pluto, the lord of the underworld, cast his amorous, roving eye on a nymphet named Mentha. His wife didn't smack him around for his infidelity but instead took it out on the nymph. She located Mentha and stepped on her so ferociously that she was trodden into the ground. Pluto, sorry at being caught in the act but still longing for Mentha, changed her into a fragrant herb so he could still enjoy her presence even with Persephone, his wife, looking on.

The herb has been used for centuries to treat digestive problems. The healing ability is concentrated in its essential oil, which contains menthol.

Peppermint oil is used in great amounts commercially for flavoring toothpaste, chewing gum, candy, chocolate, breath mints and so on.

The essence can be used safely at home to help heal indigestion, nausea and colic as well as to relieve bloating and flatulence. It is a good remedy for diarrhea and an aid to prevent morning sickness and travel sickness.

As late as 1979, doctors were still investigating the various aspects of the essential oil as it relates to the stomach. In fact, it is now recommended for the painful condition known as irritable bowel syndrome because of its antispasmodic properties. It should be noted that in a double-blind study using synthetic and natural peppermint oil, only the natural oil gave sustained relief.

Peppermint oil is an anti-inflammatory *when sufficiently diluted*; otherwise it will cause irritation and inflammation. Small amounts are stimulating while large amounts are inclined to be sedating. It is of great value as an inhalant during colds, flu or sinus congestion. Dilution is important so two or three drops of the essence in a bowl of hot water is sufficient. Use no more than two or three drops on a bit of brown sugar or in honey water for internal use.

Rose
Rosa damascena

Essence obtained from: flowers

Odor: floral

Cultivated in: Bulgaria, Turkey, Morocco

Most common uses:
　anxiety
　constipation
　depression
　emotional difficulties
　gall bladder problems
　hangover
　menstrual difficulty
　PMS
　impotence

frigidity
skin care
sensitive or aging skin

A rose is a rose is a rose. There is no known meaning for its name. Not in mythology, nor in antiquity. In all languages it's called a rose.

Early poets of Greece, China and Persia sang praises to this flower and pressed roses have been found in the tombs of Egypt . . . some still bearing traces of its delicious fragrance.

Rose essence is expensive—$655 for half an ounce—and that's too bad, because it is among the most useful of the essential oils. The other two are lavender and tea-tree oil.

The rose gives us two different extracts: the essential oil, also known as rose otto, and the absolute, which differs from the otto (which is colorless) by having an orange hue. It is the essential oil that you want to use in aromatherapy.

Bulgarian rose oil is the world's best. The roses bloom for just 30 days and must be hand-picked in the mornings only during the months of July and August. As the sun rises in the heavens, the essential oil content of the flowers drops sharply due to evaporation so the time to pick the flowers is carefully regulated. The yield is small. An experienced picker can pick 110 pounds of flowers in a day; however, 110 pounds of flowers yield only 7.5 cc of the essence.

A different species of the rose is grown in

China and has been used in medicine for 5,000 years. It has been recommended for liver, stomach and blood difficulties and it drives away melancholy.

The 17th Century herbalist Nicholas Culpeper also mentions that red roses strengthen the liver and in 18th-century Bulgaria, rose oil was prescribed for jaundice. It was also used to treat the gall bladder.

Nowadays, the essential oil is considered useful against alcoholism and the negative emotions of jealousy, envy and resentment.

Rosemary
Rosmarinus officinalis

Essence obtained from: leaves

Odor: camphoraceous

Cultivated in: Tunisia

Most common uses:
  hair loss
  mental weakness
  rheumatism
  muscular aches
  liver weakness
  gall bladder problem

Rosemary is steeped in religious tradition and stands as a symbol of fidelity and remembrance in two of the holiest of Christian ceremonies, the wedding and the funeral.

The name probably comes from the Latin *ros* meaning dew and *marinus* (of the sea) because its native habitat was the misty hills of the Mediterranean seasides.

Shakespeare's Ophelia, mourning her father's death in Act IV, Scene vi of *Hamlet*, laments:

There's rosemary, that's for remembrance;
  pray you, love remember;
and there's pansies, that's for thoughts.

Medieval herbalists thought rosemary had the power to cure nervous afflictions and even was able to restore youth.

It was prescribed inwardly for the head and heart and outwardly for the sinews and joints.

Rosemary was also the main ingredient of "Hungary Water," the first toilet water to make an impact in Europe in 1370.

According to legend, Hungary Water was invented by an old hermit to cure his queen, Elizabeth of Hungary, of paralysis of the joints. The water was prescribed to be rubbed on the sore joints. An ad for Hungary Water in the United States in the 1920s stated, "Now it is certain that rosemary has the power to increase the memory, invigorate the brain and cleanse the joints of pain."

We do know that rosemary is a nervous stimulant, a cardiac stimulant and that it improves respiration, digestion, kidney function, liver function, gall bladder function, blood circulation, and the power of the adrenal glands.

Since we know there is a strong connection in the brain between odor and memory, and that this herb is a nervous system stimulant, it's reasonable to make the connection that rosemary can stimulate the brain. So the old herbalists apparently knew what they were talking about when they said it improves memory.

Because of its stimulating effect on blood and lymph flow when applied to the skin, rosemary oil is useful for all kinds of aches or pains, whether due to rheumatism, sprains, strains or simple overexertion.

It's also claimed to be a stimulant to the scalp and to the hair follicles. This suggests that it may be the answer to baldness but there have been no double-blind studies to prove it.

Sandalwood
Santalum album

Essence obtained from: wood

Odor: musky, woody

Cultivated in: India

Most common uses:
  cystitis
  urinary infection
  throat infection
  dry skin
  autoimmune disease
  persistent infections

The Japanese remember their dead by burning incense of sandalwood. In China, sandalwood incense is burned continuously under a portrait of the deceased until the funeral. In India, it is burned at funerals and the wealthier the deceased, the more sandalwood is offered to the fire.

Lest you become depressed by the funereal connotation, Hindu holy men use sandalwood paste, colored yellow and applied to their foreheads, as a symbol of spirituality. In Hindu marriage ceremonies, sandalwood is burned and the perfumed smoke is made to waft over the bridal couple.

Sandalwood has been used in India for 2,000 years to relive genitourinary problems, while Chinese physicians prescribe it for acne, hiccups and vomiting.

The Emperor of China was so taken with the aroma of sandalwood incense that it was burned as an offering wherever he appeared and continuously in court. The demand for sandalwood eventually led to its cultivation in Lingnan Province. However, because the tree is a very slow grower, requiring some 30 years to reach 25 feet, the demand for it soon decimated the available wood. There are now very few sandalwood trees left in China and the incense has to be imported from India.

Although it has been used alone as a perfume, it is not recommended for that purpose. The sweet, woodsy fragrance is inclined to be a bit heavy. It is mainly used as a fixative in the perfume industry because it is very long-lasting.

In aromatherapy it is a useful antiseptic,

particularly for throat infections and infections of the urinary tract. It has been used as a massage, diluted, to help laryngitis.

Sandalwood oil is another one of the essences which is able to stimulate the immune system. This is important to know when the flu season rolls around. Frequent baths with sandalwood keep the immune system at peak and help prevent invasion by viruses or bacteria.

Many sources say this herbal is aphrodisiac in nature. We prefer to think of it as a sexual restorative rather than an aphrodisiac, in that it restores natural inclination as opposed to stimulating sexuality from scratch.

Dry skin and, conversely, some cases of acne respond to treatment with sandalwood essence, along with a proper diet and a gentle cleansing routine.

Tea-Tree
Melaleuca alternifolia

Essence obtained from: leaves

Odor: spice

Cultivated in: Australia

Most common uses:
   respiratory
   urinary
   dermatitis and other skin conditions
   vaginal
   insect bites and stings
   burns
   cold sores

mouth ulcers
thrush
lice
ringworm
athlete's foot
boils

This is another case of the ancients teaching the moderns. For centuries, the Bundialung Aborigines of Australia used the leaves of a particular tree as part of their medicinal arsenal. Whenever anyone in the group had skin problems or an infected wound, leaves were plucked from the tree, crushed to liberate the oil and then a poultice was made and applied to the affected area. In almost no time at all the "cure" was affected.

When Captain Cook and his crew ventured Down Under, his cook took some of the leaves to brew some tea. It was spicy and very stimulating, a pleasant change from the monotonous sea fare. That's how the tea-tree got its name.

Tea-tree grows in a relatively small, swampy region along the northern coast of New South Wales and is a member of the family which includes myrtle, clove and eucalyptus. Its odor is similar to that of eucalyptus but spicier and much more pleasing to the nose.

The tea-tree reputation appears to be too good to be true—except that it *is* true. As an antiseptic it is the most powerful of the aromatics. As early as 1925, laboratory experiments in Sydney, showed that it had an antiseptic ability that was 12 times stronger than that of the standard, which was phenol (carbolic acid). The report claimed it was unique among essential oils.

About five years later, a medical journal commented on the use of tea-tree for infected wounds. The oil cleaned the wounds without damaging the underlying tissue. Dirty wounds can be washed with a 10 percent solution to help remove debris and begin the healing process.

And in 1937, research published in *Australian Journal of Pharmacology* showed that the presence of organic matter such as blood or pus simply increased the antiseptic power of this wonder essential oil.

Australian fighting men charged into battle carrying tea-tree oil in their first-aid kits. The response was so great that demand exceeded the ability to supply the essential oil, so synthetic material was used instead. This led to a reliance on the synthetic products which was followed eventually by the increased use of antibiotics, so tea-tree oil was relegated to the back shelf.

Then, in the year 1972, a medical survey done on 60 common foot problems treated with tea-tree oil found that 58 conditions had either been completely relieved or greatly improved. The problems included corns, callouses, athlete's foot, bunions, hammerhead toes, fungal infections under the toe nail, and odoriferous feet. The athlete's foot fungus was caused by four different organisms, one of which was *Candida albicans*, yet all cases responded to the tea-tree treatment.

Ringworm is another condition caused by a fungus similar to that which causes athlete's foot. Most cases also respond to this essential oil in a few days.

In a study reported in *Obstetrics and Gynecology*, vol. 19 (6), 1962, pp793–5, the use of tea-tree oil for trichomonal vaginitis (inflammation) and other vaginal infections was discussed.

Of the 130 women who took part, 96 were suffering from trichomonal vaginitis, while others had thrush or cervicitis. Since this was a scientific study, a control group of 50 other sufferers with vaginitis was given standard trinchomonal suppositories. These are available over the counter and on prescription in drugstores.

Tea-tree oil was used diluted on saturated tampons and douches. All the women using the tea-tree oil reported a successful conclusion and the percentage of cures was the same in both groups. However, the group using tea-tree said that it had a cooling, soothing effect and was superior in alleviating the offensive odor. None of the participants using tea-tree complained of irritation or burning.

Two other studies reported on *Phytotherapie*, vol. 15, 1985, pp. 13–15, dealt with vaginal yeast infections and with chronic cystitis.

The first of these studies was on 28 cases of thrush caused by the overgrowth of the yeast *Candida albicans*.

In this study, the tea-tree oil was prepared in capsule form and inserted vaginally once at night. After 30 days, 27 of the participants were examined and 23 were completely free of the infection. Four showed moderate improvement and one had discontinued the treatment because she felt vaginal discomfort the first night.

The second study was performed with 26 female patients suffering from chronic cystitis. They were treated orally with tea-tree oil over a period of six months. Half the patients received tea-tree oil and the other half were given a placebo which had the appearance and smell of tea-tree but was a harmless and inactive substitute.

After six months, out of the 13 who took tea-tree, seven were completely cured after suffering for years. None of the control group showed any improvement.

This oil is not to be considered a cure-all and should not be taken orally except under the supervision of a health professional. But it is being increasingly used by herbalists and laypeople for cuts, wounds, ulcers, sores, boils, burns, ringworm, athlete's foot, psoriasis, impetigo, anal and genital itching, cold sores, lice, genital herpes, bad breath, mouth ulcers, and infected gums. Quite a sensational list for an oil taken from a tree!

Tea-tree is an ideal oil for the nuisance type of problems that can clog up a doctor's office and put you at risk when you go there. After all, there are more germs per foot in a doctor's office than anywhere else except maybe a hospital. Who needs it, if the condition can respond to a few drops of essential oil suitably prepared?

By the way, this substance is much stronger than the usual household disinfectants by four to five times, yet it is gentler to the skin.

Ylang-Ylang
Cananga odorata

Essence obtained from: flowers

Odor: floral

Cultivated in: Madagascar

Most common uses:
   depression
   impotence
   frigidity
   palpitations
   rapid breathing
   high blood pressure

Ylang-ylang means flower of flowers.

Although ylang-ylang has a pronounced effect upon the body systems in the physical sense, it has an even more pronounced effect upon the emotional system. In fact, it is this action for which it is most often used in aromatherapy.

The plant is native to Indonesia and the Philippines even though it is cultivated mostly in Madagascar. The tree usually reaches a height of 25 feet and bears yellow flowers. The flowers must be harvested in the morning before the sun extracts its toll on the essence. The aroma is intensely sweet and heady, and when concentrated the effect may be too strong for some people. However, when it is properly diluted or mixed with other oils, it is irresistible.

Ylang-ylang is one of the main ingredients in Macassar oil, which was popular in Victorian times because of its salutory effect on the scalp. It was because of the popularity of this pomade that anti-macassars were devised so that the oil would not rub off on the backs of overstuffed chairs.

Ylang-ylang pomade got its start in the Molucca Islands where it was mixed with coconut oil and rubbed over the entire body in winter to ward off disease. The women used it in their hair all year round as a perfume.

Jasmine and ylang-ylang are often confused even though the scents are distinctly different. Perhaps it's because these two aromatics are the best aphrodisiacs around— outside of the bark of the yohimbine tree.

The Rest of the Essential Oils

Although you will not use more than perhaps 20 different essential oils in your lifetime, it is interesting to know about the rest of the discovered oils and their properties.

Use of these essential oils should be undertaken only with the help of a professional aromatherapist or your health professional, particularly if they are to be taken internally. It takes a lot of study to understand all of the attributes of essential oils, and they might be helpful under one condition but not others.

As time passes and more people in the medical community begin to appreciate the value of essential oils, their usage will become more commonplace. Already in Europe the practice of aromatherapy is undergoing a tremendous revival.

Aniseed
Piminella anisum

Essence obtained from: seeds

Most common uses:
   antispasmodic
   stomachic
   carminative
   diuretic
   migraine accompanied by nausea
   vertigo
   painful periods
   palpitations

Anise is an old-fashioned herb with many valuable properties. It will help prevent fermentation of food in the stomach by promoting digestion. This will help to prevent the formation of gas and check griping of the bowels.

Homo sapiens is not the only species attracted to anise. Mice have such an affinity to the herb that it was used as a mousetrap bait in the 16th century. According to several old herbals, mouse found the odor irresistible.

Its licorice-like flavor has made anise a special herb in cooking cakes and soups and it is also used in beverages and medicines.

Basil
Ocymum basilicum

Essence obtained from: herb

Most common uses:
   bronchitis
   colds
   depression
   dyspepsia
   earache
   fainting
   gout
   hysteria
   insomnia
   mental fatigue
   migraine
   nausea
   nervous tension

Also called sweet basil and, in India *tulsi*, this herb is used in the ancient healing system known as ayurvedic medicine and is sacred to Krishna and Vishnu.

Basil (rhymes with dazzle) has a split personality. It is a favorite culinary herb and is found in almost every kitchen but, on the other hand, it was thought by the ancients to have awful and evil power. It was said that it could mysteriously draw scorpions to it and that it was an herb of the war god Mars, and under the Scorpion, an evil herb named *basilicon*.

The Eastern sentiment toward basil is one of unequivocal reverence. It is hailed as a protector. Sprigs of the Indian variety are placed on the breast of the dead to protect them from other-worldly evil.

Basil is native to Asia but is now cultivated in Europe, North Africa and the Seychelles. The essence derived from basil is green-yellow in color and contains linalol, which is also found in lavender and bergamot. The odor is light and pleasant; the taste is piercing and a little bitter.

According to Dr. A. Chandrashekhar, in his book *Ayurveda For You*, the juice of the leaves is to be used when a person has been bitten by a snake (1 to 2 teaspoonsful every 3 hours), can be applied to a scorpion sting, can cure an earache by instilling into the ear, and—when mixed with cinnamon and cloves, cardamom, sugar, and milk—it helps cure the common cold and influenza. The juice also serves as rejuvenator if taken twice a day at the rate of one teaspoonful.

A recipe for coughs is also given. Take the juice of the leaves with the juice of garlic and honey. It probably works by keeping people away from you thereby limiting the number of germs you could contact!

In the bath, basil essence is uplifting and refreshing but it has a strange effect on the skin—sort of hot and cold at the same time.

Basil has shown itself to be a good insect repellent, particularly against mosquitoes.

Benzoin
Styrax benzoin

Essence obtained from: gum

Most common uses:
  arthritis
  asthma
  bronchitis
  colic
  coughs
  gout
  laryngitis
  skin irritation
  sores

Benzoin is a balsamic resin obtained from trees of the genus *Styrax*. Styrax is the ancient Greek name of storax, the name applied to a sweet-scented gum and to the tree it came from. Benzoin is from the Arabic *ben*, meaning "fragrant" or the Hebrew *ben*, meaning "branch," and *zoo*, an exudation. Putting the name together you get the juice of the branch.

Benzoin was unknown to the early Greeks and Romans. It was first mentioned by Ibn Batuta, who visited Sumatra in the 14th century. In the 16th century it was considered to be a precious balsam and part of the trade of oil brought to Venice.

The tree is now cultivated in Java, Sumatra and Thailand. It is best known in the form of compound tincture of benzoin or friar's balsam. Most people are familiar with this substance, having used it at one time or another in their steam vaporizers.

The gum is not a natural product of the tree. It would not be produced by the tree if a cut in the bark were not made. The tree produces the gum to heal the wound.

Benzoin is of benefit in all cold conditions such as coughs, flu, bronchitis, stuffy nose, etc. It is also used externally in skin conditions where there is redness, itching, cracked or dry wounds.

Marguerite Maury in *The Secret of Life and Youth* recommends a blend of cinnamon and benzoin for exhaustion of an emotional or psychic nature.

Bergamot
Citrus bergamia

Essence obtained from: fruit

Most common uses:
   acne
   bronchitis
   colic
   cystitis
   depression
   dyspepsia
   eczema
   fever
   flatulence
   halitosis
   herpes
   nervous tension
   psoriasis
   skin care

stomatitis
vaginal itching
wounds and ulcers

Cultivated in Italy and not to be confused with a similar scented tree which grows in North America, true bergamot is obtained from the rind of a fruit which grew profusely around the city of Bergamo in Lombardy, Italy. The fruit looks like a pear-shaped orange and the essence is sweet and citrusy with a floral undertone, more like lavender than neroli. It is green-yellow in color with a bitter taste.

Note: This essential oil should not be applied to the skin before going out into the sun. It is considered to be phototoxic and can cause pigmentation of the skin. This negative action to normal skin has led researchers to use bergamot oil as a treatment for *vitiligo* (piebald skin).

Bergamot oil has a slightly irritating effect on the skin if used in high concentrations, but if used in dilution of one percent or less, the opposite effect is noted. Skin conditions such as eczema, psoriasis, acne and ulcers often respond to its use. It can be especially helpful when the skin condition has been brought about by stress.

It has been used with good effect and helps to ease the discomfort of chicken pox, shingles and cold sores. It is combined with eucalyptus and either alcohol or carrier oil and dabbed on the eruptions. This helps to ease the pain and speed up the recovery.

Throat and urinary infections respond well to bergamot when used in inhalation therapy, as a gargle or in a bath. Its expectorant effect is helpful in bronchitis. Simply mix with lemon essence and use as an inhalant.

Cystitis and thrush respond well to sitz baths using this essential oil.

Bergamot is also used for emotional problems. Its uplifting, antidepressant action works against tension, worry and anxiety for men and women alike.

According to the Chinese, the sweet varieties of citrus increase bronchial secretions and the sour promote expectoration. They all quench thirst and are carminative in action.

Bergamot is considered to be a citrus in China, and when combined with neroli and lavender it makes a classic *eau de cologne*. Bergamot is one of the oils used to flavor Earl Grey tea.

Black Pepper
Piper nigrum

Essence obtained from: fruit known as peppercorn

Most common uses:
   catarrh
   colds
   colic
   cough
   diarrhea
   fever

flatulence
flu
nausea
vertigo

It is not likely that you will be using much of this essential oil. It is light yellow in color and has an aroma similar to that of clove oil. The taste is hot and bitter.

The plant, cultivated widely in Malabar, Java, Sumcha and Penang, grows naturally to a height of 25 feet but is stunted for commercial picking purposes. Black peppercorns are the sun-dried red berries which are picked before ripening. White peppercorns are the same berry that has been allowed to ripen and the outer shell removed before drying.

The name pepper comes from the Latin *piper* and from the Sanskrit *pippali*, which shows you how long ago pepper was used by mankind. Records of its use go back almost 5,000 years.

In homeopathic practice, black pepper oil is used for difficulty in concentrating, headache, nosebleed, colic, flatulence, coughs, palpitations, difficult urination and a sad state of mind.

Externally, it is rubefacient (it reddens the skin as it boosts circulation) and is gently analgesic, especially good for muscular aches and pains.

Chamomile
Anthemis nobilis, Matricaria chamomilla

Essence obtained from: flowers

Most common uses:
- allergies
- boils
- burns
- colic
- colitis
- convulsions
- depression
- dermatitis
- diarrhea
- dysmenorrhea
- dyspepsia
- fever
- flatulence
- gastritis
- headache
- hysteria
- insomnia
- irritability
- menopausal problems
- migraine
- neuralgia
- rheumatism
- teething pains
- vertigo
- vomiting

The Saxons of ancient England knew chamomile as *maythen* and it is one of the oldest known medicinal herbs. Along with lavender and peppermint, it is also one of the best known oil-producing herbs in that country. Chamomile was known as the "plant physician" for its ability to treat so many conditions and because it appeared to keep other plants healthy when planted near them.

If you have to take antibiotics, it's a good idea to eat yogurt, take lactobacillus acidophilus capsules, and drink chamomile tea with milk sugar (lactose) to help restore the normal intestinal flora.

Medical interest in chamomile took a big jump when it was discovered that it contained azuline. When this compound is isolated from the herb, it takes the form of deep blue crystals. These crystals are an excellent anti-inflammatory agent and they work their magic in very small amounts. It is now being used in a number of pharmaceuticals. Azuline is not present in the fresh flower but is formed when the essential oil is distilled.

The essential oil has an odor reminiscent of apples and the taste is pleasantly bitter. When mixed with rose, geranium and lavender, it makes a refreshing bath oil.

Chamomile is good for many female disorders including scanty menstruation, painful or irregular periods, uterine hemorrhages, vaginitis and menopausal problems. It is also used for children because of its low toxicity and its anti-inflammatory action.

Mental stress, anxiety and nervousness respond well to this essential oil.

Cardamom
Elettaria cardamomum

Essence obtained from: seeds

Most common uses:
   colic
   cough
   dyspepsia
   flatulence
   halitosis
   headache
   loss of appetite
   nausea
   mental fatigue

This plant grows plentifully in Ceylon, India and China. The seeds are rather large, about half an inch long, and yield an oil with an agreeable sweet, spicy scent.

Older herbal texts say the oil is warming and comforting, helps digestion, strengthens the stomach, dispels wind, is good for colic and cold disorders of the stomach and bowels and is useful to promote urine.

Its main activity is in the stomach and it teams up with peppermint to form a workable alimentary team. This combination helps soothe the nausea of pregnancy. Like peppermint it will help you to avoid vomiting but if the stomach needs emptying it will not prevent it.

After a siege of vomiting it helps bring the body back to normal. It is used for bad breath when the cause of this condition is not from infected teeth or bad dental hygiene. (Bad breath is frequently caused by improper digestion of foods. This essential oil can help bring about normal gastric workings.)

Although primarily for the digestive system, many people find the aroma uplifting and use it to clear their minds for constructive thinking. The effect may be strictly psychological but those who have tried cardamom in an inhaler swear by it.

Cinnamon
Cinnamomum zeylanicum

Essence obtained from: leaves and bark

Most common uses:
   promotes appetite
   carminative
   antiseptic
   colds
   indigestion

The oil obtained from this plant is a yellow color which turns brown as it ages. The best oil comes from Sri Lanka although that obtained from China is almost as good.

For the stomach, combine 1 drop of the essential oil with 1 drop oil of peppermint on a little brown sugar.

For colds, use as an inhalation. Or try this recipe:
1 jigger of good whisky
½ squeezed lemon
1 tablespoon honey

Put these in a glass of hot water in which three drops of the essence has been dissolved.

Clove
Eugenia caryophyllata

Essence obtained from: flower buds

Most common uses:
   Externally for
   scabies
   infected wounds
   toothache
   mosquito repellent

Note: Clove oil can produce skin irritation if used in high concentrations on sensitive skin.

Citronella
Cymbopogon nardus

Essence obtained from: grass

Most common uses:
   insect repellent
   neuralgia
   headache
   migraine

The Chinese use it for rheumatic pain. Try a dilution of citronella on the temples to treat insomnia.

Cypress
Cupressus sempervirens

Essence obtained from: fruit

Most common uses:
   asthma
   diarrhea

dysentery
dysmenorrhea
influenza
menopausal problems
nervous tension
rheumatism
skin care
varicose veins

The cypress tree originated in the East and is commonly found in gardens and graveyards.

The oil is clear with a woodsy-spicy aroma. It is more of a masculine than a feminine scent.

It exerts action on the female reproductive system, possibly via the ovaries, and has shown its value in menstrual and menopausal disorders.

It is also a powerful antispasmodic and useful to asthmatics and those suffering from spasmodic coughing fits. A drop of cypress essence on a tissue near a sickbed can often help soothe explosive coughing.

Eucalyptus
Eucalyptus globus

Essence obtained from: fresh leaves

Most common uses:
asthma
bronchitis
burns
catarrh
cough
emphysema
fever

influenza
throat infections

This is a big tree! It can reach a height of 480 feet and is indigenous to Australia. The name comes from the Greek *eukalyptos*, meaning well-covered, because the buds are protected by a cup-like membrane. The essence has a distinct camphor-like odor and a bitter taste that feels cool to the tongue. It is a wonderful antiseptic oil probably due to its ability to produce ozone. A two percent emulsion of the essence sprayed in the air kills 70 percent of the airborne staphylocci. Note: This is a powerful essence. One or two drops in any preparation is usually sufficient.

Insects are repelled by its odor. Use 1 or 2 drops in 2 ounces of water, shake well and apply to the skin. Eucalyptus can be used effectively on animals as well as humans to repel fleas and pests.

Fennel
Foeniculum vulgare

Essence obtained from: seed fruit

Most common uses:
  alcoholism
  amenorrhea
  colic
  constipation
  dyspepsia
  flatulence
  menopausal problems
  nausea
  vomiting

Note: This essence is not to be used before exposure to the sun as it can cause skin discoloration.

This plant grows to a height of about five feet and bears golden flowers. The name is from the Latin *foenum* meaning hay. It was a favorite herb of the ancient Romans, and Pliny attributed over 20 remedies to it. In cookery, it was used to combat obesity and was said to convey strength, courage and longevity. It was also said to be helpful to the eyes.

In medieval times it was called *fenkle* and was used to ward off evil spirits.

Fennel is a good diuretic and can be used when there is a scanty flow of urine. Its action in obesity is said to be hormonal, due to its content of anethole. This indicates its use in menopausal situations.

It is of use in alcoholism since it prevents toxic build-up and expels waste material.

For internal use you can make a mixture of 1 to 5 drops of fennel essence in honey water three times a day.

Frankincense
Boswellia thurifera

Essence obtained from: gum

Most common uses:
    bronchitis
    catarrh
    coughs
    dyspepsia

    laryngitis
    skin care
    ulcers
    wounds

This herb was one of the gifts offered to the infant Jesus because it was thought to be as precious as gold.

The ancient Egyptians used it in cosmetic facials as a rejuvenating essence. It is an astringent for the skin and catarrhal conditions. It is physically and mentally soothing to asthma conditions and helps calm the panic which accompanies forced shallow breathing.

Frankincense was also known as olibanum and, along with myrrh, was among the first gums used as incense. It was first imported to Egypt from Africa 5,000 years ago. The smoke from the burning incense was used as a fumigant to cleanse the sick and to drive out the evil spirits who caused the illness. Later, it was used as a cosmetic aid and rejuvenating element in clay masks.

Geranium
Pelargonium odorantissimum

Essence obtained from: the whole plant

Most common uses:
    burns
    depression
    dermatitis
    diarrhea
    eczema

nervous tension
neuralgia
shingles
skin care
stomatitis
wounds

In the folklore of Islam, geraniums were said to be a gift from Allah. As the legend goes, Mahomet went bathing one hot dusty day, leaving his shirt on a clump of weeds. When the prophet came out of the water and picked up the shirt, the weeds had been transformed into geraniums.

Native Americans used geraniums to treat a wide variety of medicinal conditions including cholera, gonorrhea, neuralgia, toothache and as a styptic on open wounds.

The essence is clear to light green and has a sweet fresh scent. It makes a very refreshing and relaxing bath oil. It mixes well with rose, citrus oils and basil but it can go with almost any other essence. In spite of its lovely color and delightful scent, geranium has a bitter taste.

It is a mild analgesic and sedative and may be used for neuralgia and pain that comes from nerves. It is an excellent remedy for burns and is renowned for its efficacy on ulcers and wounds.

The action of geranium on the nervous system is both sedative and uplifting, like bergamot, and is useful in helping to alleviate anxiety states. Like basil and rosemary it is a stimulant to the adrenal cortex whose hormones are essential to balance hypersecretion of either androgens or estrogens, such as often occurs during the menopause.

Because of its terpene content, geranium can act as an insect repellent without repelling your friends.

It is a useful essence for all types of skin conditions including eczema, shingles, ringworm and lice infestation. It is also of great value in skin care for almost any type skin. It is a cleansing, refreshing, astringent and mild skin tonic. Geranium essence can also be used if the skin is inflamed and sensitive.

Hyssop
Hyssopus officinalis

Essence obtained from: herb

Most common uses:
  amenorrhea
  asthma
  bronchitis
  bruising
  catarrh
  colic
  cough
  dermatitis
  dyspepsia
  eczema
  flatulence
  hysteria
  otitis
  rheumatism

Hyssop hides among other plants in dry, hilly places. It is a small herb, only one to two feet in height, with pointed leaves and flowers of a pale blue hue. It likes a warm and dry climate. Its small size hasn't interfered with its value in aromatherapy and it is mentioned in the Bible as one of the aromatic herbs.

The essential oil is golden-yellow in color and is one of the herbs which gave the cordial Chartreuse its characteristic color and flavor. Its odor is hard to describe because it is unlike any other. It smells like a mix of basil, thyme and geranium. The effect, however, is not difficult to qualify: a feeling of alertness and clarity, a clearing of mental debris.

Note: Hyssop essence is contraindicated for those suspected of suffering from epilepsy.

Hyssop is a stimulating oil with an unusual effect on blood pressure. It tends to regulate pressure, raising it if it is low or lowering it if it is too high. It is also very helpful to the respiratory tract, helping to liquify mucus and to relieve bronchial spasms. It is an excellent cough remedy and can be of benefit in asthma, bronchitis, influenza, and the like.

Applied externally, hyssop helps heal bruises and soothes the scaly skin of eczema sufferers.

Jasmine

Jasminum officinale, j. grandiflorum

Essence obtained from: flowers

Most common uses:
   anxiety
   cough
   depression
   frigidity
   impotence

This is an expensive essence, so when you use it, enjoy it! In China, it is used largely to scent tea, to decorate women's hair and to massage the body after bathing. All three uses are worth it because it has an exquisite scent.

The oil is a deep red-brown. Jasmine blends well with rose and with citrus oils to make fascinating combination aromas.

Jasmine's main thrust is to the emotions and it is of exceptional value when applied to psychological and/or psychosomatic ills. It calms the nerves and at the same time lifts the spirits. It is an antidepressant and can produce a feeling of optimism and confidence.

Along with its sister essence, the rose, jasmine affects the female reproductive system. It can help to relieve uterine spasms and menstrual pain. It is also considered an effective aphrodisiac, warming and relaxing the body. Because of this and because it affects the emotional sphere, jasmine is considered to be an asset in treating impotence or frigidity. It is also active on the male libido and sexual organ in a warming and strengthening manner.

Jasmine is helpful to the respiratory tract, relieving cough, nervous spasms in the throat and bronchial passages, and difficulty in breathing.

Juniper
Juniperus communis

Essence obtained from: fruit berries

Most common uses:
   acne
   amenorrhea
   colic
   cough
   cystitis
   dermatitis
   dyspepsia
   eczema
   flatulence
   gout
   hemorrhoids
   skin care
   urinary tract infections
Note: Juniper should be avoided during pregnancy and by those with kidney disease.

Gin makes a good aperitif because juniper is one of the important ingredients and it is an appetite stimulant.

Juniper is a small evergreen tree, usually four to six feet in height. The berries look like black currants and turn from green to black-purple as they ripen. The best oil comes from the berries. A cheaper, less potent oil can be obtained from the branches but it has less therapeutic value.

Juniper was used in Tibet in ancient

times for religious and medicinal purposes. It was mixed with rosemary (twigs of jupiter and leaves from rosemary) and burned in hospitals to purify the air during epidemics.

The oil has a tinge of green-yellow color to it and a turpentine-like odor which is pleasant. Like the pine and cypress, it makes a refreshing bath oil and is both relaxing and stimulating at the same time.

Juniper oil acts on the skin, digestion, nerves and on the genitourinary tract as a diuretic. It is also a good antiseptic to these areas. Some people use juniper for gout and rheumatism.

Juniper is also a good remedy for colic and flatulence. All minor stomach disorders and digestion could benefit from the use of this oil.

Lemon Grass

Cymbopogon citratus

Essence obtained from: grass

Most common uses:
  stress-related conditions
  muscle aches and pains
  deodorant
  insect repellent

Most people are not crazy about its odor— and neither are ticks and fleas. It has been used in Indian medicine for centuries in spite of its extremely strong odor. Lemon grass is found in Brazil, South Africa and Sri Lanka, where it is combined with neroli and used as a calming agent for stress-related diseases such as colitis.

In a massage oil, it can ease muscular problems and the aches and pains of too much exercise. Combine it with rosemary for the best effect.

Research done in India shows that lemon grass essence acts as a sedative on the central nervous system, so three drops diluted with a carrier oil in a bath can be sedating and refreshing as well as deodorizing.

This oil has a strong antiseptic, bactericidal and antifungal effect in proper dilution.

Lemon
Citrus limonum

Essence obtained from: fruit

Most common uses:
   infections
   debility
   dyspepsia
   colds and flu
   skin conditions
   insect repellent
   to protect the vascular system
   thrush
   otitis
   wounds
   nosebleeds
   tonsillitis

To lose weight, try pouring a cup of boiling water on two heads of chamomile and one sliced lemon. Leave the water sit overnight and then drink the first thing in the morning. It will stimulate bowel action and suppress appetite.

The fruit is used in a number of preparations or the essence itself can be expressed from the outer part of the fresh rind. Green fruit will yield more essence than ripe fruit. The essence contains terpenes, citral, citronella, aldehydes and lemon camphor.

Marjoram
Origanum marjorana

Essence obtained from: herb

Most common uses:
  arthritis
  asthma
  colds
  colic
  constipation
  dysmenorrhea
  dyspepsia
  flatulence
  headache
  hypertension
  hysteria
  insomnia
  migraine
  nervous tension

The ancient Greeks used marjoram in medicine, perfumes and cosmetics. In medicine it was a remedy for convulsions, dropsy and narcotic poisoning. The essence has a very bitter taste but, when mixed with lavender and bergamot, makes a pleasant and relaxing blend. In the bath it is relaxing and warming.

Marjoram oil is stimulating to the parasympathetic nervous system, resulting in a general vasodilation. It is an excellent addition to a body massage oil. Marjoram is warming and analgesic and so it helps in muscle spasms, strains, sprains, rheumatism and so on.

A bad cold can be helped by the use of marjoram in an inhalation therapy.

Mandarin
Citrus reticulata

Essence obtained from: peel

Most common uses:
   general tonic
   digestive stimulant
   intestinal problems
   nausea

This is the tiny orange you find in supermarkets, usually canned and under the name Mandarin orange. It got its name because it was a traditional gift to the Mandarins of China. Its gentle action makes it particularly suitable for children's upset stomachs. Also, the scent is immediately soothing.

To prevent stretch marks during pregnancy, combine
1 drop mandarin
1 drop lavender

1 drop neroli
¼ ounce almond oil
½ tsp wheat germ oil

Massage skin gently from the fifth month onward.

The same formula can be used to soothe children's tummy aches. Apply and massage in a clockwise direction.

Melissa
Melissa officinalis

Essence obtained from: herb

Most common uses:
  allergy
  asthma
  colds
  colic
  depression
  dysentery
  fever
  indigestion
  hypertension
  menstrual problems
  migraine
  nausea
  nervous tension
  vertigo

The leaves of melissa have an oil which resembles lemon oil and the aroma is very much like that of lemon. There is no botanical relation between the two but they do resemble each other.

The name comes from the Greek word for honey, because any bees will make a beeline for the melissa flowers in their vicinity.

It is one of the earliest medicinal herbs, highly esteemed by Paracelsus, who called it the elixir of life. Its action is tonic and anti-spasmodic rather than stimulant. It slows respiration and the pulse, lowers blood pressure and relaxes smooth muscle.

Melissa seems to have an affinity for the female reproductive system. It has a mild emmenagogic action (that is, it helps promote normal menstruation) and is useful for painful periods. This is due to the relaxing, antispasmodic action. It is also helpful in menstrual irregularity and female infertility because its relaxing action permits nature to function at her own rhythm.

Its activity on the digestive tract resembles that of peppermint. It relieves spasms, permitting a normal flow of digestive juices. It is used to treat nausea, vomiting and indigestion, particularly when these conditions are of nervous origin. Also, it is good to relieve flatulence.

Orange Blossom/Neroli
Citrus vulgaris

Essence obtained from: flowers

Most common uses:
    depression
    chronic diarrhea
    hysteria
    insomnia

nervous tension
palpitations
shock
skin care

A rose is a rose is a rose, but this is not so of oranges. There are two types of orange tree, the sweet orange, *Citrus aurantium*, and the bitter orange, *Citrus vulgaris*. Oil of orange blossom, usually called neroli, is extracted from the white blossom of the bitter orange tree. Strangely, the fruit is not used.

The blossom of the sweet orange also yields an oil but it is of inferior quality and not used at all in aromatherapy.

The name is thought to come from a princess of Nerola who crushed the flowers to scent her gloves. She was a trendsetter, the wife of a famous 16th century Italian prince, and her practice was duplicated. At one time, gloves scented with neroli were known as *guanti di neroli.*

Bitter orange is not native to Europe but was probably introduced by Portuguese sailors from the East Indies. The tree is a native of China where it has been used for medicine and cosmetics for centuries. It is now cultivated in France, Tunisia, Italy and the United States.

Although the essence is most commonly thought of as a component of eau-de-cologne (combined with lavender, lemon, bergamot, rosemary), the classic toilet water, it is one of the most effective sedative/antidepressant oils.

The oil is a pale yellow in color with a bitter taste and a sweet, feminine odor. It helps calm the mind and relieve spasms, hence its use for palpitations. Its calming action also indicates its use for panicky, hysterical or fearful types of people.

Neroli can help to relieve the effects of shock and conditions resulting from long-standing stress.

Like lavender and geranium, neroli can be used on all skin types. It is soothing and can even be used when the skin is irritated or red. It is one of the oils which can act cellularly, stimulating new skin growth and elimination of old, dry skin.

In the bath, neroli is relaxing and deodorizing. A skin treatment and a mental treatment at the same time.

There is a mixture called orange flower water that is soothing, digestive, carminative when used internally. It can be used for infant's colic and it also promotes sleep.

When there is trouble in our stress-filled world, reach for neroli. It is one of the most precious buffers for stress-related problems, shock, hysteria, worry, fear, nervousness, panic. Any thoughts which are disturbing sleep patterns will respond to neroli. It calms and soothes the mind, the body and the spirit.

Patchouli
Pogostemon patchouli

Essence obtained from: herb

Most common uses:
  anxiety
  depression

skin care
wounds

Before "I Go Pogo" there was pogostemon, known as *puchaput* in India. The flowers are white and purple. The Paisley weavers of Scotland copied Indian designs but couldn't sell their merchandise because it didn't "smell right." Once the printed shawls were scented with patchouli they were accepted in the worldwide market.

Patchouli oil gets better with age so don't throw it out after six months' sitting. It has a deep red-brown color and its scent has been compared to the odor in a musty attic or that of a coat hanging in that attic. Crueler people have said it has a goat-like aroma. It is an excellent fixative when combined with rose, yielding an exquisite, long-lasting scent.

Patchouli is also reputed to be an aphrodisiac but you'll have to prove that for yourself.

People used to say that every part of a pig was useful except the oink. Now, every part of a plant is useful—including its fragrance.

Plants are the lungs of the world. They take in the carbon dioxide we breathe out and give us oxygen. They provide us with food, beauty and healing. Plants are miracles.

This book is not the definitive study of essential oils. Those that have been mentioned have a history of usage, but as research continues and the use of essential oils enters the mainstream of medicine, we shall find that nature has given us one more priceless tool.

Glossary of Terms

absolutes—perfect, complete, whole; in this sense, the final result (the concentrated essential oil) which is obtained after extraction of delicate flowers by the enfleurage method. It takes a tremendous amount of flowers to yield absolutes of rose and jasmine, for example, which is why they are very expensive. However, because they are highly concentrated, only a miniscule amount is needed.

alcohols—colorless, pungent liquids that form esters when they react with organic acids; sometimes used as a solvent in extracting essential oils

alopecia—baldness or loss of hair on the head through illness, heredity or age

amenorrhea—abnormal absence or suppression of menstruation

analgesic—a substance that takes away pain without affecting consciousness. Analgesic oils that are often used with compresses are lavender and chamomile.

anoint—to massage or rub

antiseptic—something that prevents infection, kills germs; or something that is free of infection, sterile

antispasmodic—a substance which relieves involuntary muscle contractions or cramps.

Examples include lavender, marjoram and clary sage.

aromatherapy—the practice of using the essential oils of plants for healing. The term is believed to have been coined by Rene-Maurice Gattefosse in 1937.

aromatic—of or having an odor or aroma; something that smells sweet, spicy, pungent or fragrant. Each component of an essential oil is an aromatic chemical.

aromatic baths—baths in which oils are used for health or cosmetic purposes. Depending on the essential oil used, aromatic baths can be refreshing and stimulating or relaxing and sedative. Add the essential oil to a vegetable base, then add to the bath water, stirring the water by hand to help disperse the drops of oil.

astringent—something that contracts blood vessels and body tissue, checking the flow of blood; or having a harsh or biting quality. Essential oils with this quality include chamomile, frankincense and sage.

Bach flower remedies—developed by a Welsh physician, Edward Bach, in the 1930s, they are a system of 38 self-help remedies made from flowering trees, bushes, and wildflowers. They aim to treat the mental or emotional state behind physical ailments. The premise is that, by allowing patients to find their own peace of mind, the remedies help people heal themselves.

Some aromatherapists recommend the Bach flower remedies in conjunction with their own treatments.

bacteracide—something that kills bacteria or germs. Essential oils that are bactericides include eucalyptus, thyme and tea-tree.

base oil—the principal or essential ingredient; or the one acting as a vehicle for the essential oil, which is very rarely used full strength. In aromatherapy, base or carrier oils are usually good quality cold-pressed vegetable oils such as grapeseed oil, which is odorless and thus very suited to combining with essential oils.

carminative—something that causes gas to be expelled from the stomach and intestines, such as caraway, chamomile, thyme and spearmint oils

carrier oil—see base oil

catarrh—an inflammation of the nose and/or throat which produces excess mucus. Sandalwood oil is often used to treat this condition.

chakras—the Sanskrit term for the seven energy centers of the body along the spinal column; each represents an area of consciousness. Chakras are sometimes referred to in connection with aromatherapy massage.

cold-pressed—an essential oil obtained by crushing the plant or part of the plant to extract the oil, which is then filtered.

There is no heating involved at this first-pressing stage, which produces "virgin" oil.

compress—a pad of folded cloth that is moistened or medicated and applied to a part of the body for healing, pressure, or to warm up or cool down that area.

cytophylactic—a plant product that encourages the production of new skin cells, such as frankincense

decongestant—a treatment or medication that relives congestion, especially in clogged nasal passages. Essential oils that are effective decongestants include cypress, lemon and sandalwood.

diffuser—an apparatus that diffuses an essential oil, i.e., spreads it evenly throughout the room

distillation—a method of obtaining an essential oil by steaming a large vat of plant material at high pressure to separate it. Then the vapor of essential oil and the steam are cooled, condensed and collected, to obtain a concentrated, purer form. This is the method used for extracting most true essences.

dropsy—an old-fashioned term for edema or swelling

dysmenorrhea—difficult or painful menstruation

effleurage—a Swedish massage technique

often used by aromatherapists. Slow, long, gentle strokes are made with the entire hand, always in the direction of the heart. Lighter effleurage strokes affect the nervous system, while deeper strokes are used to treat the muscles and aid circulation.

emollient—something that softens or soothes when applied to the skin

enfleurage—the method of extracting perfumes by pressing flowers in odorless fats to absorb the exhalations or essential oils. Flower heads are replaced continually as they wilt, until the fat is saturated with the blooms' essential oil. The result is called a pomade.

essential oil—a highly concentrated, aromatic extract of a single plant, whether a flower, seed, fruit peel, grass, leaf, tree or root. Essential oils are aromatic substances that are extracted from one source through expression, distillation or solvent extraction. They evaporate easily and have a limited shelf life.

expectorant—an agent that causes phlegm or mucus to be expelled from the respiratory tract.

expression—squeezing. This is the method used to obtain the essence of most citrus oils, including lemon, mandarin, bergamot, orange and lemon. Oil droplets are expressed or squeezed out of the peel of the fruit.

extraction—to obtain essential oil as an extract by distilling, pressing or using a solvent

fumigation—to use fumes or smoke to disinfect or kill bacteria

fungicidal—something that checks the growth of spores, molds or fungi

hypertension—high blood pressure

hypotension—low blood pressure

infused oil—an essential oil obtained by steeping or soaking so as to extract the essence. In ancient times, infused oils were obtained by soaking plant material in a base of vegetable oil, then sitting it in the sun or heating it.

infusion—the fluid extract that remains after steeping something in water, alcohol or other fluid.

inhalation—the act of inhaling or taking in a vapor, which gets the oil into the bloodstream through the lungs. Inhalations of essential oil mixtures are usually recommended to treat the lungs or respiratory system.

leukorrhea—an abnormal, whitish discharge from the vagina

limbic system—the part of the brain which is linked to emotion, memory, and contains olfactory nerve tracts maceration—to separate by steeping in fluid (oil)

meridians—energy lines in the body, according to acupuncture, often followed in shiatsu, a Japanese form of massage

oil burner—a device which slowly diffuses essential oil into the air to freshen a room, promote sleep or relaxation (lavender), or act as a bactericide in a sick room (eucalyptus)

organic solvent—solvents used to extract essential oils from flowers

perfume—in ancient times, these were good-smelling fluids that were almost 100 percent composed of aromatic essences. Today synthetic aromatic chemicals are used to produce perfumes and scented cosmetics, which is why they have none of the therapeutic effects of essential oils. However, the most expensive perfumes usually contain as much has 20 percent of an essential oil.

phenols—a dilute solution used as an antiseptic

pheromones—a hormone secreted by animals and humans that evokes a response, in this sense, an attraction response

photosensitization—becoming sensitive or reacting to light; phototoxic. Certain essential oils are sensitive to ultraviolet light and should not be used on the skin before you spend time outside because they will cause pigmentation of the skin.

phytotherapy—literally, plant therapy, using plant material to heal

pomade—a thick oil or perfumed ointment applied to the hair to groom it; the fatty mixture that is saturated with essential oils after the first stage of the enfleurage method

pressure extraction—a method of obtaining essential oils by squeezing the plant or flower

pruritis—intense itching of the skin

reflexology—foot massage based on the theory that the area on the bottom of your feet can be divided into different zones that are related to and refer to different parts of the body. Massage in these areas is used to help heal and prevent distress in the part of the body that corresponds to that zone. Occasionally it may be used as part of aromatherapy treatment, but probably only as a diagnostic tool.

rubefacient—a reddening agent, or something that stimulates the circulation, thereby causing that area to redden

shiatsu—a Japanese type of massage based on ancient Oriental theories about meridians (lines of energy) in the body. The meridians and pressure points that are treated are the same ones referred to in acupuncture.

solvent extraction—a way of extracting or obtaining the essential oil of a plant or flower by using either benzene, butane, alcohol or luxane (solvents). A very large amount of macerated flowers is then soaked in a solvent. This mixture is then put through a centrifuge to separate the waxes and oils from the solvent and scrap material. Next the oil and wax solids are distilled, and lastly, the wax is separated from the absolutes, that is, the final result. This process is very expensive and time-consuming, so it is used primarily for flowers such as jasmine and roses, which are too delicate for the distillation process.

stomachic—an old-fashioned term for a substance which aids digestion, such as spearmint, peppermint and tangerine

unguent—oil

vaporization—to change something into a mist or steam (vapor) suspension in the air, by spraying or heating to evaporate. Vaporization of essential oils can create or change a mood in an environment, or be used to fight infection, depending on the oil selected.

vermifuge—a drug used to expel worms or parasites from the intestines

virgin oil—the highest quality oil which is extracted from the first pressing of the plant material

zone therapy—see reflexology

Resource Guide

This information is provided as a service to our readers only, and is not intended as a personal endorsement. Also, since the field of aromatherapy is growing rapidly in the U.S., there may be more sources of products than we can include here; this guide should not be considered all-inclusive.

Aromatherapy Associations

The American Aromatherapy Association (AATA) sponsors annual conventions, has referral lists of practitioners available, and is promoting industry regulation and recognition of aromatherapy and the essential oils.

American Aromatherapy Association
3384 South Robertson Place
Los Angeles, CA 90034
800-869-9514

National Association of Holistic Aromatherapy (NAHA)
P.O. Box 17622
Boulder, CO 80308-7622

In England, you can contact:

The Association of Tisserand Aromatherapists
44 Ditchling Rise, Brighton
East Sussex 8N1 3PY
England

Or you can try:

International Federation of Aromatherapists
46 Dalkeith Road, Dulwich
London SE 21 8LS
England

For more information about the practice of aromatherapy, including courses of education and/or referrals to aromatherapists in your area who have completed those classes, contact the American Aromatherapy Association at the address given above.

The AATA offers weekend and two-day seminars for beginners (laypeople interested in discovering more about this fascinating field) as well as advanced training classes of six days. The Association has also developed a computer software program titled "Aromatherapy Treatment and Blending Program" for practitioners.

The teachers include Marcel Lavabre, the founder and president of the AATA, and Michael Scholes, an aromatherapist.

AIR
P.O. Box 12021
Fair Oaks, CA 95628
(916) 965-7546

Courses in holistic aromatherapy are taught by aromatherapist Victoria Edwards of NAHA.

Esthetec
580 Lancaster Avenue
Bryn Mawr, PA 19010
(215) 525-7516

Courses on aromatherapy for aestheticians are offered on a regular basis by Kay Acuazzo.

National Association of Holistic Aromatherapy (NAHA)
Address and telephone number on page 193.

Holistic aromatherapy is taught by aromatherapist Ann Berwick, through a correspondence course which emphasizes theory and a one-week hands-on practical course followed by an internship. The course includes a study of the essential oils, their properties, their effects on body systems, energetic aromatherapy, aromatherapy massage, facials and lymphatic drainage and consultation techniques. The course is directed at practitioners and a certificate is given upon satisfactory completion of the entire course.

The Pacific Institute of Aromatherapy
P.O. Box 903
San Rafael, CA 94915
(415) 479-9121

Kurt Schaubelt, Ph.D., a chemist and doctor of natural sciences from Munich, Germany, heads the Institute, and helped found the AATA, of which he is vice president. The Pacific Institute of Aromatherapy concentrates more on the academic and scientific aspects of aromatherapy, including extensive research into ethnobotany, popular science, plant pharmacognosy and the preparation of data for medical journals. The Institute's correspondence course, the International Certification Course in Aromatherapy, is scientifically based and is five years old, and experts from the Institute are available for lectures and seminars. Referrals are given to naturopaths who are versed in aromatherapy techniques as well as naturopathy.

Sources of Essential Oils

(Check also with your local health store.)

Aroma Vera
3384 South Robertson Place
Los Angeles, CA 90034
800-669-9514

The Aroma Vera line of aromatherapy products was developed by Marcel Lavabre and uses pure essential oils and natural carriers exclusively.

Essential oils are available in bulk to distributors and retail outlets, as well as to individuals who can order by mail. Aromatic diffusers, books on aromatherapy and information on seminars are also available from Aroma Vera. Anyone interested in or considering using essential oils may call this toll-free number and ask for their free catalog.

Aveda Corporation
400 Central Avenue Southeast
Minneapolis, MN 55414
800-328-0849

The Aveda Corporation was founded by world-renowned hairstylist and photographer Horst Rechelbacher, who created its aromatherapy line of hair, skin and body care products after his own health crisis led him to investigate holistic healing and wellness philosophies. The products are made from whole herbs and pure ingredients as they are found in nature. Rechelbacher believes that environmental harmony starts from within, through a holistic approach to nutrition, cleansing, exercise and nourishment of the mind as well as the body. The product line is available through several dozen distributors across the U.S. who supply the aromatherapy products only to salons and spas with a staff trained by Aveda in the use of the essential oils. For the name of a salon featuring Aveda products near you, or if your business is interested in featuring the Aveda line, call the toll-free number.

Beauty Klinick
3268 Governor Drive
San Diego, CA 92122
(619) 457-0191

The Beauty Klinick is a day spa and health and beauty institute catering not only to beauty needs but also to health and balance of the mind, including stress relief and reduction. President and Founder Linda-Anne Kahn is a specialist in aromatherapy and lymphatic drainage, as well as having credentials in massage, skin care and nutrition. The Klinick offers clients a full range of pure essential oils, including bath oils, skin care oils and lotions blended with them to suit clients' needs, whether it be cleaner skin or a stress-reducing soak.

Desert Essence
P.O. Box 588
Topanga, CA 90290
(213) 455-1046

This company offers a line of body and skin care products made with tea-tree oil.

Euro Health & Beauty, Inc.
6555 No. Powerline Road, Suite 404
Fort Lauderdale, FL 33309
(305) 938-7513, 800-783-7369

This firm offers equipment and its own line of products catering to the spa, salon and aromatherapy trade, including natural body and skin care products, hydrotherapy tubs, Moor Mud, essential oils, etc. Spa and salon consulting is also available. Referrals are given to people outside the trade interested in armomatherapy and purchasing essential oils. Elisabeth Devaud is the vice president; her articles on phyto-aromatherapy have been published in the quarterly journal of the AATA.

Leydet Oils
4611 Awani Court
Fair Oaks, CA 95628
(916) 965-7546

Original Swiss Aromatics
Pacific Institute of Aromatherapy
P.O. Box 903
San Rafael, CA 94915
(415) 479-9121

Pure essential oils are sold to practitioners and distributors wholesale and through mail order.

Preferred Source
3637 W. Alabama, Suite 310
Houston, TX 77027
(713) 662-2190

Wild or organic essential oils, aromatic diffusers, bath oils and body oils are available. They offer the Aroma Vera line of products which was developed by Marcel Lavabre.

Quintessence Aromatherapy Inc.
P.O. Box 4996
Boulder, CO 80306
(303) 258-3791

Pure essential oils and select blends are available for sale.

Essential Phyto Aromatics
Time Laboratories, Inc.
P.O. Box 3243
South Pasadena, CA 91031
(818) 300-8097

Essential oils in their own line are 100 percent pure and natural. They also offer skin care products and bath oils that are blends of aromatherapy oils; their products are distributed to aromatherapists through Time Laboratories and other distributors.

True Essence Aromatherapy
1910 Bowness Road, N.W.
Calagary, Alberta T2N 3K6
Canada
(403) 283-5653

Wild or organic essential oils, aromatic diffusers, bath oils and body oils are available. They offer the Aroma Vera line of products which was developed by Marcel Lavabre.

Whole Spectrum
Essential Products of America, Inc.
5364 Ehrlich Road, Suite 402
Tampa, FL 33625
800-822-9698

Whole Spectrum has over 100 unadulterated true essential oils in stock, as well as certain blends for massage, bath and facial use. They provide an analysis of every oil sold to consumers and offer a money-back guarantee of satisfaction.

Publications About Aromatherapy

Aromatherapy Quarterly was established in 1983 in England by Tricia Davis, the author of *Aromatherapy: An A to Z.* American readers can subscribe for one year by using a MasterCard or VISA card. Contact: Aromatherapy Quarterly, 5 Ranelagh Avenue, London SW13 OBY, England.

Common Scents is the quarterly journal of the American Aromatherapy Association. Nonmembers of the AATA may subscribe at a cost of $20 for four issues: 3384 South Robertson Place, Los Angeles, CA 90034.

Scentsativity is a quarterly journal published by the National Association of Holistic Aromatherapy and is available to members of NAHA. For more information, write to P.O. Box 17622, Boulder, CO 80308-7622.

Bibliography

Chandrashekhar, *Ayurveda for You.*

Lautie, R. and A. Passebecq, *Aromatherapy.* Thorsons Ltd., Wellingborough, Northamptonshire, England, 1984.

Lavabre, Marcel F., *Aromatherapy Workbook.* Inner Traditions Publishing, Vermont, 1988.

Lee, William H., *Herbs and Herbal Medicine.* Keats Publishing, Inc., New Canaan, Connecticut, 1982.

Martin, Gill, *Aromatherapy.* MacDonald & Co. Ltd., London, 1989.

Maury, Mme Marguerite, *The Secret of Life and Youth.* Thorsons Ltd., Wellingborough, Northamptonshire, England, 1990.

Price, S., *Practical Aromatherapy.* Thorsons Ltd., Wellingborough, Northamptonshire, England, 1985.

Tisserand, M., *Aromatherapy for Women.* Thorsons, Ltd., Wellingborough, Northamptonshire, England, 1985.

Tisserand, Robert B., *The Art of Aromatherapy.* Destiny Books, Rochester, Vermont, 1977.

Tyler, V. E., L. R. Brady, J. E. Robbers et al., *Pharmacognosy* (Eighth edition). Lea & Febiger, Philadelphia, 1981.

Valnet, Jean, *The Practice of Aromatherapy.* Destiny Books, Rochester, Vermont, 1978.